THE EASY A
COC

70+ Delicious Recipes to Prevent and Heal Acid Reflux Disease & GERD

ADELE LORAIN

SUMMARY

Introduction 1

Chapter 1: Does your heartburn? 7

   1.1 Avoid top offenders 15

   1.2 Lighten up 22

   1.3 Trim down Portion Sizes 26

   1.4 Make Light Meals a Daily Affair 31

Chapter 2: Don't stop Eating 42

   2.1 Aim for a healthy weight 53

   2.2 Don't Have Too Much Alcohol 58

   2.3 Follow a Low-Carb Diet 64

Chapter 3: Making life Tasty 73

   3.1 The Pros and Cons of Acid Reflux 86

   3.2 Light Food Healthier Life 97

   3.3 Enjoy Eat Travel 111

Chapter 4: Managing Your Meals and Trigger Foods 131

   4.1   Steps and Precautions 142

   4.2 Best Drinking Practices 149

   4.3 Holistic Dietary Plans for GERD 157

   4.4 Foods to Eat for Evading Acid Reflux Every day 158

   4.5 Natural Remedies 174

Chapter 5: Your food, your healer! 187

   5.1 Sore Throat and Acid Reflux 198

   5.2 Pregnancy and Heartburn 206

Conclusion 215

References 219

Introduction

Acid reflux is a common condition in the lower chest with a burning pain called heartburn. When acid returns to the food tube, it happens. Gastro esophageal reflux disease is treated more than twice a week when acid reflux occurs. While specific statistics vary, acid reflux disorders are the most common bowel condition among hospital departments in the United States. Acid reflux usually leads to heartburn, whether because of a GERD episode that is overwhelming or chronic.

Heartburn is a gross sensation of discomfort that is felt behind the esophagus. It seems that lying down or bending down is getting worse. After eating food, it can take several hours and sometimes worsen.

Heartburn pain can go up to the neck and stomach. In certain situations, the fluid of the stomach may enter the back of the mouth, giving a bitter or sour taste.

When heartburn happens twice a week or more, it is immediately known as GERD. Heartburn is also known as acid reflux, indigestion, or pyros. This occurs when some acidic stomach content returns to the esophagus. Acid reflux causes burning pain, often after feeding, in the lower chest area. Lifestyle risk factors include obesity and smoking. The most common drug treatments are available on prescription and counter therapy.

Severe, repeated cough and wheezing are some symptoms of GERD. Asthma and persistent pneumonia can also be found. Nausea with Ailment and Throat distress, such as soreness, heaviness and laryngitis (voice box inflammation), Chest or upper abdominal pain. Dental loss, poor breathing without treatment, GERD, can lead, including an incrustation, to serious longer-term consequences.

The U.S. College of Gastroenterology reports about 60 million People experience heartburn once a month and 15 million at least as many times as daily. It is the most popular among western countries with an estimated 20-30 percent of the population. Chronic cardiovascular disease can cause severe complications. Persistent exposure to stomach acid may cause esophageal damage, leading to the inflammation of the throat skin that in some cases causes irritation, bleeding and ulceration. Damage caused by acid in the stomach adds to the scar preventing the swallowing of food trapped in the esophagus. A substantial problem of esophagus reproduction. This is why it is generally recommended to have a full acid reflux control system with the aid of appropriate and monitored meals. A proper dietary routine will lead the person to recovery without the natural and healthy use of medicines. By taking yourself on board and disposing of waste from your life, you can enjoy and live every minute with healthy food full of flavor, using the recettes that will be addressed in future chapters according to different tastes and food combinations recommended by nutritionists worldwide.

Acid reflux happens when some acid content of the stomach goes into the esophagus, into the throat and forces food down from the mouth. Heartburn, despite its name, is not something connected to the heart. This contains hydrochloric acid, a strong acid that helps to break down food and to protect it from bacterial pathogens. The lining of the stomach is particularly designed to protect it from strong acid, but does not protect the esophagus.

A muscle ring, the esophagus gastrointestinal sphincter, usually serves as a valve that enables food to reach the stomach, not the esophagus. When that valve fails, signs of acid reflux, such as heartburn, are felt and the stomach material is revitalized to the throat. This affects individuals of all ages. It is often because of a lifestyle aspect and unhealthy dietary habits without meals. It can also be because of triggers that cannot always be avoided.

A hiatal hernia (or hiatus) is one because it cannot be prevented. A depression in the diaphragm emerges into the top of the uterus, which rarely reaches the chest cavity. Certain risk factors are easier to control: obesity, smoking (active or passive), lower exercise levels, drugs like asthma, calcium blockers, antihistamines, painkillers, sedatives, and antidepressants Acid reflux may also be caused by pregnancy because of extra pressure on internal species.

It can be prevented by maintaining a healthy lifestyle, which controls the entire reflection mechanism with a nutritionally controlled diet, meal schedules and eating procedures.

Food and acid reflux dietary habits include: heavy caffeine use, excessive alcohol consumption, high salt levels in food. A diet that contains low dietary fibers. It can also be a reason to lie down immediately after eating a meal and having large meals. Eating large amounts of chocolate, carbonated drinks and acid juices.

Another study suggests that dietary options may be as effective as using injury care proton pump inhibitors.

Including diet and regular meals, Zantac is one drug for heartburn relief.

Pipes, including omeprazole, rabeprazole and esomeprazole, are the first treatment options for acid reflux. H2 antagonists include cimetidine and ranitidine. Over-counter drugs, such as antacids, which can be purchased online. Alginate medications like Gaviscon are either pipes or H2 tubes, both of which are drugs, the primary treatment choice for patients with chronic GERD acid reflux. Such medications are usually safe and effective, but are not suitable for all reflux patients, such as any prescription medication. You may have side effects. A proper dietary balance shall be maintained in conjunction with such medications.

For example, they may cause nutrient absorption problems. This could lead to malnutrition. Antacids provide quick, but short-term relief by reducing acidity of the stomach.

These include chemical compounds such as calcium carbonate, sodium bicarbonate, arsenic and magnesium hydroxide. These can also inhibit nutrient absorption, leading to deficits over time.

Other possible treatment approaches include: potassium-competitive acid blocker foods, low transient esophageal sphincter stimulation (TLESR), GABA(B) receptor agonist, antagonists Mglur5, Prokinetic agents, Stress modulators, tricyclic antidepressants, selective serotonin reuptake inhibitors (saris) and Theophylline. Specific treatment methods included: Apart from salts, habits require steps that facilitate the completion of acid reflux and meals. Strengthening posture or sitting straight, Using loose clothes and Weight loss if obese or overweight. Stop increasing pressure on your belly, such as tight belts or sit-ups. Stop smoking Acid reflux can cause lower chest burning pain.

Chapter 1: Does your heartburn?

When stomach acid flows into the food pipe, heartburn happens. This creates an intense burning sensation in your abdomen that can move up to your throat and back. You may have a bitter or sour taste in your throat back too. Heartburn lasts from a few minutes to several hours, and will often feel worse after feeding.

Occasional heartburn is frequent, and over-the-counter antacids can usually alleviate this. Acid reflux, gastro esophageal reflux (GERD), indigestion of acid, and reflux are also known as the condition.

You may get gastro esophageal reflux disease (GERD) if you have heartburn often, and it is severe. If so, speak with your doctor.

What do you think of heartburn?

Heartburn signs include:

A burning sensation in the chest happens after eating and lasts for a few minutes to several hours. Chest pain, particularly when leaning over, lying down or feeding

Burning in the throat. Warm, bitter, acidic or salty-tasting fluid at the back of the throat

Trouble swallowing. A sense of "sticking" food in the center of the throat

Some factors can cause heartburn or make it feel worse. These include:

Eating habits

Eating large portions of food. Eating certain foods such as chocolate, peppermint, citrus fruits, spicy foods, and tomatoes or tomato-based products. Drinking alcohol, citrus juices, coffee beverages, and carbonated beverages. Eating shortly before bedtime.

Lifestyle habits

Changes in diet and lifestyle can prevent and manage your heartburn. The first things to try are:

Don't walk to bed with a full stomach. Eat at least three to four hours of meals before you lie down. This allows emptying the stomach and reduces the chance of heartburn.

Don't over-consume. Reduce portion sizes at mealtimes, or serve 4 or 5 small meals instead of 3 large ones.

Slow eat. Remember to place your fork between bites. Wear loose-fitting clothes.

You may want to find other approaches that you can use to eliminate foods and drinks that trigger your symptoms of heartburn. Write down the meals in a heartburn diary, which seems to cause your discomfort.

Shed several pounds to relieve symptoms. Follow a Healthy Weight Loss Plan if you are overweight. Halt cigars. The lower esophageal sphincter (or LES) may be damaged by nicotine. This muscle regulates the space between the stomach and the esophagus. The LES prevents stomach contents containing acid from entering the esophagus.

Elite beer. Try exercise, walking, meditation, stretching, or deep breathing instead of drinking to relieve stress. Drink hot liquids, for example, herbal tea.

Keep track of when heartburn hits and the specific activities which tend to cause accidents. What is a keen home cook to do? The challenge is even harder because there is no single food or type of food that can be labeled "heartburn food." Some people get heartburn from citrus, a symptom of gastro esophageal reflux disease (GERD). Others have problems consuming alcohol or coffee. For some people, even chocolate can cause heartburn.

And a particular ingredient that upsets someone after one meal can cause after another no problems at all. Still, a few tips will help you serve a safe, nutritious, heartburn-friendly meal afterward that will not leave your family and friends suffering.

RECIPE#1 GARLICKY OLIVE, WALNUT, AND EDAMAME MIX

Total Time: 10 min Prep Time: 10 min Cook Time: 0 min Servings: 8 (1/2 cup each)

Nutrition Highlights (per serving):155 calories13 g fat 7 g carbs 6 g protein. At each party, you'll always find a group of people socializing by the food table, mixing in a snack mix without a thought. Treat your guests with this savory and balanced garlic olive, walnut, and damage blend. Its low-carb and protein packed. Plus, the leftovers, if any, make a quick snack which is easy to pack!

Ingredients:

- 1 cup of walnuts, toasted

- 1 cup of calamite olives, pitted

- 2 cups of frozen shelled damage, defrosted

- 1 teaspoon of extra virgin olive oil

- 1/2 teaspoon of garlic powder

- 1 tablespoon of fresh rosemary leaves

10

Directions:

1.   Toss all ingredients together.

2.   Serve straightaway. Refrigerate any remainders.

To keep it interesting, you may use a mixture of different olives. Try Castelvetrano olives with a mild, smooth, buttery flavor, briny and bitter Nylon olives, or fatty and oily Nicosia olives. A tip for those who struggle to eat attentively: use olives that still have the pit. This slows down and enjoys the aromas, so that you don't accidentally swallow a hole! Just as in this recipe you can use different types of olives, so you can use different kinds of nuts as well. If allergic to tree nuts, try these at most well stocked grocery stores with pumpkin seeds or even crunchy roasted chickpeas that you can make yourself or buy. Make this more delicious by adding a crunchy or flaky sea salt sprinkle that adds texture and adds even more flavor. If you're making a bigger batch, you might want toast your nuts in the oven. Spread them on a baking sheet flat, and toast for about 10 minutes at 400 degrees. They might also be toasted over medium heat in a dry skillet, sometimes tossing to avoid burning.

Whatever method you use check your nuts frequently as nothing will ruin this recipe more than the bitter taste of an excessively toasted nut. This recipe uses only a tablespoon of rosemary, so you're sure to have some leftovers. Apply it to a chicken or pork marinade and add lemon juice, garlic, sugar, and mustard. Or sprinkle it over roasted potatoes and cauliflower. It's a beautiful, sturdy herb, so leftover rosemary is well stored in the freezer too.

RECIPE#2 COD PARCHMENT PACKS

Cooking in parchment is still a trendy cooking technique—who doesn't want to make and clean dinner with handy and elegant paper packages at the same time?

Cooking in parchment is a low fat, simple and effective form of cooking where steam aids cooking, so you don't have to add extra oil. The lower-fat aspect makes this dish free of worries for those experiencing heartburn. Pile in protein, veggies, and herbs and in minutes a complete meal is ready.

Ingredients:

- 2 cups of sweet potato, julienned
- 1 pound of cod, cut into 4 parts
- 1 teaspoon of dried thyme leaves
- 4 teaspoons of olive oil
- 1 teaspoon of kosher salt
- 4 slices of fresh lemon Directions:

Directions:

1.   Oven preheats to 400F.

2.   Fold into half 4 sheets of parchment paper.

3.   on one side of the parchment, place 1/4 of the sweet potatoes and top with a piece of cod.

4.   Sprinkle with 1/4 teaspoon thyme, 1 teaspoon of olive oil, 1/4 tablespoon, salt and a slice of lemon

5.   Fold the parchment paper over the fish and vegetables to create a closed and crescent-shaped bundle.

6.   Package a baking sheet to bake for 20 minutes.

7.   Remove from the oven, and allow for 5 minutes of rest before opening.

8.   Replace cod with other options for low fat seafood such as tilapia, shrimp or flounder. These are all choices made for high quality protein.

Try thin strips of other nutrient rich veggies, such as carrots, butternut squash, or zucchini, instead of sweet potato. All three of these are kind to heartburn.

Citrus fruit like lemon can be problematic for heartburn (it's a known heartburn trigger), but fish and olive oil mellow the small amount in this recipe. For those with heartburn, switching out low pH foods to achieve a more neutral pH in the final dish is actually a standard useful tip.

Alternatively, just use the lemon zest. Make sure all the skin has been removed from the fish; ask your fishmonger to do that for you.

Use kitchen shears for easy opening of parchment packets when ready to serve. Let steam escape, and then serve on large plates.

1.1 Avoid top offenders

Great list of foods that cause heartburn. But a few foods stand out as natural causes for heartburn. These include onions, tomato sauces, orange, chocolate, and mint sauces. If someone is suffering from acid reflux in your household, try avoiding these things. Watch then to see if doing so provides relief from heartburn. Traditional fatty foods such as bacon or ham can be replaced with oatmeal, fresh fruit, and perhaps a little pint of cinnamon for flavor for breakfast.

Oatmeal contains a high content of fiber, which promotes healthy bowel habits, reduces portion size, and also tastes good. Cereal with milk and fresh fruit will provide an attractive breakfast alternative to fatty meats. Melons are also good at preventing heartburn since they are only mildly acidic while giving a snack or meal that is filling, water-rich, and nutritious.

Whole grain bread may be toasted or topped with fresh fruit, small quantities of eggs, nut butter, or yogurt for another healthy but appealing meal. Also, rice or couscous is the right choice, mainly brown rice, which is rich in fiber. Fresh bananas are a significant natural element for preventing acid reflux, as they have very little acid content. They coat the esophagus ' mucous lining and thus reinforce mucosal defenses against reflux. The fiber in bananas also accelerates the passage of food through the gut, preventing food stasis in the stomach for longer than necessary, thereby limiting acid production, while reducing the chances of acid reflux. Eat bananas, pineapples, or other non-citrus juices at breakfast. Offer the tea as a coffee alternative. Check out non-tomato casseroles, lasagna, homemade pizza, and other main course recipes. For example, a great pasta sauce is made from pesto or olive oil combined with parsley and garlic. Serve fruit slices or fruit ices for desserts instead of chocolate-rich items.

RECIPE#3 BANANA GINGER ENERGY SMOOTHIES

Ingredients

- 1/2 cup ice

- 2 cups of milk

- Two bananas, ripe

- 1 cup of yogurt

- 1/2 tsp. Fresh ginger, peeled

- And 2 tbsp. fine grated honey or brown sugar (optional) Directions

Directions:

1. Add the ice, milk, yogurt, bananas, and ginger to a blender.

2. Mix until smooth.

3. Add sugar whenever needed.

RECIPE#4 DIY BAGELS

This skinnier recipe comes in a much more reasonably sized package with everything you love about bagels. It is much easier to make do - it-yourself bagels than you might imagine. Take some staples from the pantry, and bake. Saving calories and weight loss will relieve heartburn symptoms and lower the risk of chronic illness. A straightforward win - win is to switch to the home-made version.

Ingredients:

- 1 and 1/2 cup of water warm
- 1 packet of dry active yeast
- 1 cup of granulated sugar
- 3 1/2 cups of bread flour
- 2 cups of kosher salt

Directions:

1.   Whisk warm water with yeast, and sugar in a medium bowl; set aside for 10 minutes.

2.   Combine flour and salt into the bowl of an electric mixer equipped with a dough hook.

3.   Add the yeast mixture to the meal and mix for 6 to 8 minutes at medium speed, until the dough has formed into a large, smooth ball.

4.   Transfer dough into an oiled bowl (for this, coconut oil works well).

5.   Cover a clean dish towel and allow for an hour or so to rise.

6.   boil water in pot, preheat oven to 425F, and line with parchment paper on two sheet panes.

7.   Move the dough to floured surface and divide it into 8 bets of equal size. Roll dough into a ball, and poke a hole in each section with your fingers; set aside and repeat with the remaining portions of dough.

8.   Reduce heat to a simmer until water is boiling.

9.   Working in lots, put 3 bagels in the water and cook for one minute each side. remove the bagel from the water, and then place it in the prepared sheet pan.

10.   In a small bowl, mix egg and 1 tablespoon of water, and whisk well. After boiling all the bagels, brush with wash the egg. 11. Bake bagels until brown in golden color. Allow to cool, before serving for at least 10 minutes.

11.   After any of your favorite bagel flavorings have been brushed with egg wash top. Store bagels for up to one day in plastic bags. Slice and freeze fresh bagels in a safe freezer bag and place the frozen bagels in the toaster when they are ready to enjoy.

RECIPE#5 MUSELI STYLE OMELETTE

Ingredients

1 cup instant oatmeal

1 cup of milk

2 tbsp. Rosins (boiled, drained)

1/2 banana,

1/2 golden apple diced, sliced, diced

Salt 2 tsp.

shake. Sugar or Sweetheart

Directions

1.   Mix the oatmeal, milk, raisins, salt, and sugar (or honey) in a bowl on the evening before (or at least 2 hours before).

2.   Cover and put in the fridge.

3.   Also, add fruit before serving.

4.   If the mixture seems hard, add milk.

1.2 Lighten up

Fatty foods will increase the risk of heartburn as they take longer to digest, stay in the stomach and bring more upward pressure on the valve that leads to the esophagus,' the question is Tell Me What to Eat If I Have Acid Reflux?

Bake or broil food, rather than fry.

Try substituting low-fat yogurt in recipes, which include cream. Split meat portions into casseroles and stir-fries, and add more vegetables.

Use whole grains in place of refined grains, such as brown rice or quinoa. The added fiber in itself is healthy and can make a meal more filling with less fat and fewer calories.

How to savor a meal?

Fresh herbs or herbal blends may be used to add flavor to these products. If spices trigger acid reflux, they should be used in tiny amounts. Instead, they may choose herbs such as basil, parsley, and oregano.

When a sauce is requested, a low-fat recipe should be used. Herbs, cheese, nuts, and a splash of oil will create a tasty dressing that will not cause acid reflux or exacerbate it.

Is yogurt the right choice?

Not too sour yogurt is also suitable for acid reflux, thanks to probiotics that help normalize bowel function. Yogurt also provides protein and relieves the discomfort of the stomach, often providing a sensation of cooling.

Selecting foods can be accessible by looking at them to see how acidic they are. The higher a food's pH, the more likely it is to soothe your malaise. Therefore, any food with a pH greater than 5 or 6 is generally good for people with acid reflux.

RECIPE#6 GALA APPLE HONEYDEW SMOOTHIES

Ingredients

2 cups of honeydew melon (peeled, seeded, chunks cut)

4 tbsp. New aloe Vera, removed skin

1 Gala apple (peeled, cored, half cut)

1/16 tsp. Lime zest (use the zest grater)

1 and 1/2 cups of ice

1/4 tsp. SALT

Directions

1.   Add the melon, sugar, aloe Vera, mango, salt, and lime zest to a blender.

2.   Start blending on Pulse before shifting to Medium. Stop and stir the mixture to a smooth consistency as needed.

RECIPE#7 POTATOES WITH SESAME SEED

Ingredients:

3⁄4 cup instant polenta or cornmeal

3 cups of whole milk

3 tbsp. Vanilla extract

1 Tsp. brown sugar.

A 1⁄2 tsp. orange extract

1 tbsp. of salt to taste.

Directions

1.   Add Sesame Seminars

2.   Put the milk to a boil.

3.   Remove the meal of polenta or maize, and whisk vigorously to prevent lumps.

4.   Cook until smooth.

5.   Just before eating, add the sugar, salt and vanilla, and the orange extract.

6.   Serve with sesame seeds and sprinkle in a bowl.

1.3 Trim down Portion Sizes

Perhaps reducing portion size is the most effective way to prevent heartburn. The more significant the meal, the higher the risk of reflux. Creeping up in the kitchen is easy for the portion sizes. Magee recommends:

Use the measuring cups to limit how much you are cooking.

Dine on smaller plates, so it still looks a lot less like that.

Go over quantity for strength. For example, if you love chocolate — sometimes referred to as a heartburn trigger — you prefer little use of dark chocolate instead of a large dessert of chocolate.

How should they cook vegetables to prevent acid reflux?

Vegetables also taste better when roasted rather than steamed or boiled. The roasting allows the emergence and caramelization of natural sugars in those foods. Some plants that can be cooked include carrots and sweet potatoes, squash, cauliflower, and broccoli. Other methods to make vegetables taste great are to broil, sauté, or grill them, thus avoiding sharp, pungent spices during the process. The plants typically have low acid content.

Raw vegetables are also beautiful in the form of a salad. These provide nutrition while soothing the stomach. Unlike processed foods, these typically lack any added substances such as spices or salt excesses. A delicious salad, combined with chicken or beans, is easy to put together for a filling meal, which would significantly reduce the chances of triggering acid reflux.

RECIPE#8 CALM CARROT SALAD

Ingredients

1 lb. Carrots (peeled, cut and grind)

1/4lb. 2 Tbsp. muscling greens.

2 Tbsp. raisins.

1 Tsp. of orange juice.

Dried 2 tbsp. oregano

2 Tsp. brown sugar.

A 1/4 tsp. olive oil.

SALT

Directions:

1.   Blend the raisins, orange juice, oregano, brown sugar, olive oil, and salt in a dish. Let them sit for 5 minutes.

2.   Pour over the carrots to the dressing and thoroughly blend.

3.   Season with extra salt, if necessary.

4.   Serve over leaves of a muscling.

RECIPE#9 WATERMELON AND GINGER GRANITE

Ingredients

3 cups of seedless watermelon juice (blended)

1 cup of water

1/2 cup of honey

One whole clove

One teaspoon of ground nutmeg

1 tsp. Clean salt

1 tsp of ginger.

1/2 tsp. Lemon zest

Directions:

1.   Bring to a boil the water, honey, clove, nutmeg, ginger, salt, and zest for lemon. Enable, then pressure, to cool.

2.   Pour the sugar into the juice of the watermelon.

3.   Place the juice in a bowl that you can place in the freezer and freeze for 3 hours. Remove with a sauce whisk every 15 minutes.

RECIPE#10 CREAMY HUMMUS

Ingredients:

1 can (19 oz.) canned chickpeas (drained and washed twice)

1 cup stock

2 tbsp. Sesame oil.

A 1/4 tsp olive oil.

1/2 tsp. Salt

Directions:

1.   In a food processor, put the chickpeas and add the chicken stock, olive oil, sesame oil, and salt.

2.   Continue until smooth.

3.   Chicken stock should be added as appropriate.

4.   Serve cold with toast points, oven-toasted corn chips, or tiny flat-bread wedges.

1.4 Make Light Meals a Daily Affair

Experiencing heartburn isn't uncommon, especially after eating spicy foods or a big meal. Approximately 1 in 10 people feel heartburn at least once a week, according to the Cleveland Clinic. One in three experiences this every month.

If you experience heartburn twice a week or more, then you may have a more severe condition known as GERD. It is a digestive disorder that causes stomach acid to re-enter the throat. Frequent heartburn is one of the common symptoms, which is why a sour or bitter taste in the throat and mouth frequently follows the burning sensation.

Why is heartburn after eating occurring?

It passes down your throat when you swallow food and through your esophagus on the way to your belly. The swallowing action causes the muscle to open, allowing food and liquid to move into your stomach, which controls the opening between your esophagus and stomach, known as the esophageal sphincter; the muscle would otherwise remain tightly closed.

If this muscle does not close appropriately after swallowing, your stomach's acidic contents may travel back up to your esophagus. This is called "reflux." Stomach acid also enters the lower part of the throat, contributing to heartburn.

Easing heartburn after eating is a necessity, but it doesn't have to be an inevitable result of getting heartburn. Some steps can be taken to soothe the heartburn feeling after a meal. To relieve the symptoms, seek the following home remedies.

Wait for Lie down after a big meal; you might be tempted to collapse on the couch or go to bed after a late dinner. Nonetheless, doing so can lead to heartburn beginning or worsening. If after a meal you feel tired, keep active by moving about for at least 30 minutes. Try to wash the dishes, or go for a walk at night.

Also, finishing your meals at least two hours before lying down is a good idea, and avoiding eating snacks right before bed.

Wear Loose Clothing Tight belts, and other restrictive clothing can put pressure on your abdomen, which can lead to heartburn. After a meal, lose any tight clothes or turn into something more comfortable to avoid indigestion.

Don't hit 60 seconds for a cigarette, alcohol, or HEALTHLINE caffeine tool. Smokers may be tempted to have a cigarette after dinner, but it can be expensive in more ways than one. It also encourages heartburn by relaxing the muscle, among the many health problems that smoking can cause, which usually prevents stomach acid from returning to the throat.

The role of the esophageal sphincter is also negatively impacted by caffeine and alcohol.

Raise your bed's head. Try elevating your bed's head from the ground about 4 to 6 inches to prevent heartburn and reflux. When the upper body is lifted, gravity makes returning to the esophagus less likely for stomach contents. It's important to note that the bed itself, not just your head, must be raised. Providing extra pillows puts your body in a bent position that can increase your abdomen's pressure and aggravate symptoms of heartburn and reflux.

You can raise your bed by placing 4-to6-inch blocks of wood firmly at the top of your bed under the two-bed posts. You can also put these blocks between your mattress and box spring to lift your body from the knees upwards. You might find uplifting bricks in medical supply stores and some drug stores.

A further practical approach is sleeping on a unique wedge-shaped pillow. To prevent reflux and heartburn, a wedge pillow slightly elevates the head, shoulders, and torso. You can use a wedge pillow while you're sleeping on your side or back without causing tension in your head or neck. Most of the pads on the market grow from 30 to 45 degrees or from 6 to 8 inches at the tip.

Overeating will lead to too much. That increases pressure on the upper stomach valve. You are eating just before bedtime often contributes to the danger of reflux because your stomach will still be full when you lie down. Drinking water will help to dilute the stomach acids and reduce the risk of reflux. Water can also soothe the burn by washing stomach acids out of the esophagus when heartburn happens — Elite carbonated water. Carbonized water can increase pressure in the stomach and cause belching. Belching causes the valve to open at the top of the stomach, which increases the risk of acid reflux and heartburn. Start meals at home early enough to allow the gastroenterologist at Stanford University three hours before bedtime— plenty of time for the stomach to clear its contents.

Encourage family members to get up after a big meal and move instead of stretching out onto the sofa. Being upright helps prevent refluxing food. Also, a brisk walk around the neighborhood instead of half an hour of TV can help control your weight, another meaningful way of putting out the heartburn fire.

RECIPE#11 FLAVOURFUL CANTALOUP GAZAPCHO

Ingredients

1 lb. (2 cups) 2 tbsp. of cantaloupe (skin removed, seeded, cut into 1 "pieces).

Brown sugar or 2 tbsp. agave sugar

Port wine

Nice grated nutmeg dusting

Directions

1.   Mix together the cantaloupe, the sugar and the port. Put in the freezer approximately 4 hours.

2.   Blend into a mixer.

3.   Top off with a nutmeg dusting.

4.   Serve in a shot glass or a small cup straight away.

RECIPE#12 BLACK BEAN AND CILANTRO SOUP

Ingredients

Canned black beans

1-pint fresh cilantro

1/2 cup of chicken stock

1 tbsp. of salt.

nonfat crème

Directions:

1.   Bring a boil with the chicken stock. Stir in the beans, cilantro, and oil.

2.   Cook over low heat for 30 minutes.

3.   Blend into the desired consistency with a hand blender.

4.   Season, as required.

5.   Serve in a bowl of soup, and garnish 1 tsp — a sprig of cilantro and nonfat sour cream.

RECIPE #13 QUICK BANANA SORBETS

Ingredients

3 cups of seedless watermelon juice (blended)

1 cup of water

1/2 cup of honey

One whole clove

One teaspoon of nutmeg

1 tsp. salt

1 Tsp fresh ginger.

1/2 tsp. Lemon zest

Directions:

1. Put to a boil the tea, sugar, clove, musk, ginger, salt, and lemon zest. Enable, then pressure, to cool.

2.   Pour the sugar into the juice of the watermelon.

3.   Place the juice in a bowl that you can place in the freezer and freeze for 3 hours. Remove with sauce whisk every 15 minutes.

RECIPE#14 CROCKPOT CHICKEN AND BARLEY STEW

It's simple and makes the night a little less wild. Putting everything in the crockpot and turning it on. It is also very adaptable, so feel free to adjust the seasonings to suit your taste, to include herbs on hand or to avoid specific triggers

Ingredients

2 chicken breasts

3/4 cup barley

48 oz. Chicken broth, low-sodium

1 16 oz. Bag of frozen mixed vegetables 1/4 tsp garlic powder*

1 small chopped onion*

2 teaspoons Italian seasoning)

2 bay leaves Pepper to taste

Salt to taste

2 cups of chopped baby spinach

Directions

1.   Put everything in the pot except the spinach, making sure it's all covered with chick broth.

2.   Place the crockpot on the cover, set it to low and cook for 5-6 hours until the barley is tender. For the last 30 minutes add the spinach. Remove leaves from the bay and discard them.

3.   Remove the breasts from the chicken, shred and then combine with the soup

If fresh onions or garlic cause your heartburn symptoms, try substituting dehydrated onion and garlic powder for those products. Some people think that they are more tolerable. Or completely omit the onion and garlic this is a very forgiving dish.

RECIPE#15 LIGHT AND FLUFFY ANGEL FOOD CUPCAKES RECIPE

These are made from only egg whites, flour, and sugar; angel food contains zero grams of fat per serving, so they are less likely to fire up heartburn. Serve with typically heartburn-friendly fruits, such as melon, bananas, peaches, or strawberries.

Ingredients:

- 1/2 cup of cake flour and granulated sugar

- 1/4 cup of powdered sugar

- 1/4 teaspoon of kosher salt

- Six large egg whites (room temperature)

- 1/2 teaspoon of tartar cream

- 1 teaspoon of vanilla extract

Directions:

1.   Oven preheats to 350f.Line a paper-lined cupcake pan; set aside. Sift the rice, powdered sugar, and salt in a medium bowl.

2.   Place the egg whites in a separate bowl and beat them with an electric mixer until they start thickening.

3.   Add tartar and vanilla cream and beat for a further 2 minutes or until stiff peaks begin to form.

4.   Pour in sugar slowly and continue beating on high until all the sugar is incorporated. Switch off the mixer and fold the flour mixture gently, using a rubber spatula, into egg whites.

5.   When appropriately blended, spoon evenly into cupcake plate. Baking until the tops become slightly golden and the cupcakes come out clean with a toothpick from the center.

It's hard to come up with fat-free cupcakes without artificial ingredients, and this recipe couldn't be easier to make — you probably have all the ingredients in your kitchen right now. Use this cake mix in your favorite recipes instead of traditional cupcakes, or shortcake. But doesn't worry if you can't find cake flour; just combine seven all-purpose flour tablespoons with one cornstarch tablespoon. The end product gets precisely the same taste and bake. The egg whites should be treated at room temperature for the best results; this will help make the extra cake light and airy. To ensure even cooking of cupcakes, use an ice cream scoop or a small measuring cup to measure batter inside the pan. Serve with a powdered sugar dusting, a dollop of softly whipped cream and diced strawberries, or frosting whisk.

Chapter 2: Don't stop Eating

That condition will affect your entire life if you suffer from chronic heartburn that may be associated with gastro esophageal reflux disease (GERD). Stop eating some of your favorite foods may need to. The heartburn will affect your sleep. It may even compete with your flexibility to function well. But for all the food you want to have, there is no need to compromise. Just when you and your doctor agree on your GERD medication, understanding what to do is also crucial. Large meals stretch your stomach and raise upward pressure against the lower esophageal sphincter (LES), which can contribute to heartburn. Eat six smaller meals each day, rather than three bigger. This will help to keep the stomach from getting too full and will also help prevent excessive stomach acid production. Three smaller dining options and three snacks will help.

Consider these tips to stay healthy by having your favorite food:

Don't Eat Too Quickly

When we eat too quickly, it's more difficult for our digestive system to perform the way it should. We may end up suffering from poor digestion, which makes you more likely to experience heartburn. While eating, some way to help you slow down are to: Put your fork or spoon between bites. Chew the food thoroughly before you drink. Chew twenty times, or count to twenty before crack. Crunch smaller.

Don't consume the things that can trigger the heartburn

There are a few explanations why some foods cause heartburn: If the lower esophageal sphincter relaxes when it shouldn't; or if the stomach generates too much acidity.

Foods that may promote acid production and increase heartburn include: Caffeinated beverages, Carbonated beverages, Tobacco, Spicy foods, Citrus fruits and juices (e.g. you have to know what to ask for, and what to avoid. You will prevent heartburn when you see how the food is being cooked, avoid some drinks and monitor portion sizes. What to look for and ask when in a restaurant:

White meat

Lean meat cuts

Broth-based soups

Steamed vegetables

Baked potatoes with low-fat salad dressing

43

Low-fat or non-fat salad dressings

Lighter desserts, such as angel food cake

Don't smoke

If you smoke, you should consider quitting. Smoking can cause many health problems and one can cause heartburn. This is especially true of GERD people. Increased saliva production Saliva is alkaline, so it can help neutralize stomach acid. Increased saliva production Saliva can help to prevent stomach acid. Species can also alleviate heartburn by soaking the esophagus and washing it back to the stomach, thus reducing the symptoms of acid reflux ate in the esophagus.

Stomach acid changes Smoking will increase the quality of gastric acid. It can also encourage the bile salts from the intestine to the stomach that are harmful to acids in the stomach. Impairs Lower Esophageal Sphincter Functioning Smoking may weaken and relax LES, which is a valve at the junction between the esophagus and the stomach. If the LES does not function properly or relax improperly, the contents of the stomach can reflux back into the throat. Damage to the Esophagus Smoking will damage the esophagus directly, making it even more vulnerable to further injury from the acid reflux.

Don't wear clothes that are too tight

Clothes that fit tightly around the abdomen, like tight belts and waistbands, can squeeze the stomach and force food on the LES. This may cause reflux of stomach contents into the esophagus.

Don't Get Too Stressed

Stress hasn't been shown to cause heartburn. However, it can lead to behaviors which may trigger heartburn. Routines are disrupted during stressful times, and you may not be following your healthy meal, exercise, and medication routines. Because your stress can lead to heartburn indirectly, it is essential to find ways to alleviate stress, making stress-related heartburn less likely.

RECIPE#16 CHEESY CAULIFLOWER CAKES

Nutrition Highlights (by serving): 127 Calories 5 g fat 13 g carbs 8 g protein

Want to eat more cauliflower but not sure what to do with it? Even if you think cauliflower isn't for you, these tasty cakes are a must-try recipe. Boil, steam, sauté or roast the cauliflower ahead of time for extra fast meal preparation, and serve the cakes for a light and satisfying meal with salad or a piece of fish. Cauliflower and lower-fat Parmesan cheese are generally well tolerated by those experiencing heartburn because they are baked rather than fried. Any excessive grease, then. Servings: 4 (2 cakes each)

Ingredients:

2 cups (cooked)

1egg (beaten)

1/2 cup (grated) Parmesan cheese

1 cup panko breadcrumbs

Directions:

1.   Oven preheats to 375 F.

2.   Line a parchment-papered baking sheet. now Combine cauliflower, potato, cheese, and brown crumbs in a large bowl. Mash ingredients until well-mixed with a fork.

3.   They turn into 8 cakes using clean hands. Place cakes on the prepared baking sheet and spray cooking spray to the tops.

4.   Bake until golden, for 20 minutes. Before serving allow to cool slightly.

If fresh cauliflower cannot be available on your local market, use frozen as it is just as nutritious as it is new. If you are using frozen, simply thaw for 2 to 3 minutes in the microwave on high. Drain well before combining with other ingredients to remove any excess liquid and then allow cooling slightly. These are flavorful as they are but by mixing in a handful of fresh herbs such as parsley, basil, or chives, you can add an extra dimension of flavor. Broil before removing from the oven, to make the tops of these cakes extra crispy. if you choose to broil to make sure they don't burn.

RECIPE#17 PAN SEARED TILAPIA

It's common knowledge that doctors recommend two portions of fish a week to help maintain good health, and this GERD-friendly recipe is a great way to help achieve that objective. Tilapia is a mild whitefish flavor which is an excellent source of lean protein, magnesium, vitamin D and good fatty omega 3 acids. We sautéed the fish in olive oil for this dish, which only takes minutes, and then we finished it with delicious ginger mixed with pineapple, red pepper and cucumbers. Serve it with some long grain rice on the side and for a busy weeknight you will have a quick and easy meal. Healthy and friendly too!

Ingredients

1 cup long grain rice

2 TBSP grated ginger

2 Tsp. Honey

2 TBSP olive oil

1 pound fresh or canned pineapple pieces

One small English cucumber, chopped

1/4 cup chopped red sweet pepper*

1 Tsp. Olive oil

Filets

Directions

1. Cook rice as directed per package

2. Add salt and pepper

3. to combine the next four ingredients. Throw in bits of pineapple, cucumber and pepper

4. In a nonstick pan, heat 1 tsp of olive oil over medium heat

5. Tilapia filets are seasoned with salt and pepper, around 1/4 tsp per

6. Add to pan and cook 2 to 3 minutes per side 7 for about.

Nutritional information per serving: 485 calories, 2.3 g sat fat, 325 mg sodium* sweet red peppers should not cause acid reflux, particularly with this minimum amount (1/16 cup per serving).

RECIPE#18 APPLE-BERRY SMOOTHIE

If you want the sweetness of the berries tries a tart apple variety such as

Granny Smith or Pink Lady. But if you wish to the primary ingredient to be a sweet apple, try Gala or Fuji.

Ingredients

1 cup of orange juice

Four large apple peels

1 1/2 cup of frozen mixed berries

1 cup of honey

Directions

Process orange juice and apple peel in a blender for 30 seconds or until smooth. Add iced mixed honey and fried berries. It takes 15 seconds to process.

Makes four servings

RECIPE#19 BANANA WALNUT MUFFINS

This sweet treat is great for on-the-goo breakfasts. The next time you have bananas that saw better days, try a bunch!

Ingredients

2 cups Total wheat flour for 1 t.

1 1/2 t salt

3/4 cup baking powder

1/3 cup sugar

Oil (usually used coconut oil)

2 eggs

3 very ripe bananas,

1 t fork mashed.

1/2 c vanilla extract.

Chopped 1/2 c walnuts.

Non-sweetened grated coconut

Directions

1.   Oven should be preheated to 375 degrees and grease a cupcake liner with muffin tin or line.

2.   Mix the dry ingredients together.

3.   Beat the eggs and whisk in the oil and mash bananas.

4.   To the dry ingredients add the banana mixture and stir until mixed.

5.   Remove the cinnamon, coconut and walnuts and mix gently.

6.   Spoon the batter into the muffin tins, filling out around two-thirds of each compartment.

7.   Bake the muffins for 17-19 minutes until the inserted toothpick in the center of a muffin comes out clean.

8.   Remove the muffins from the oven and give them time to stand in the panatelas 5 minutes before moving them to a refrigerating rack.

Nutritional data (per muffin): 218 calories, 9 g fat, 23 g carbohydrates, 3 g protein, 139 mg sodium, 18 muffins.

2.1 Aim for a healthy weight

Sometimes it's not the quality of the food — it's the quantity. Even if you follow the rules and stay away from foods that tend to aggravate your acid reflux, you might well find that your symptoms are still furious and fast. This could be because you are not looking at the amount of food you eat. The more you eat, the more your stomach will be paid, and the longer your stomach will be churning away. Eating small meals in the day and eating light at night is a perfect way to eat for many health reasons (better for diabetes, obesity, etc.), so you can add reflux of acid to the list now. There is a food move to liberty dedicated only to this novel and healthy way of eating. If your bedtime is 11 p.m., then the last dinner call should be 7 p.m.

Late evening meals are a problem. Lying down soon after you have eaten or drunk asks for trouble. Purely physical explanation. When you're standing or sitting up, your stomach is upright and the contents of your stomach must work against gravity to spray your esophagus upwards

When lying down or reclining, the stomach contents automatically churn against the valve separating the upper abdomen from the lower esophagus, as the gravity does not hold it back anymore.

So, ensure that your last meal always leaves the stomach when you're about to go to sleep, stopping eating or drinking for at least three or four hours until you lie down.

This means that if bedtime is 10 p.m., the last dinner call should be at around 6 p.m. While we're at it, it's also a good idea not to exercise vigorously soon after eating, especially bending or running activities — it also encourages refluxing.

Lying down with a full stomach causes stomach contents to press harder against the lower esophageal sphincter, increasing the chances of refluxed food. Follow these tips:

Wait to go to bed for two or three hours after eating.

Stop snacking in late at night.

If one of your meals ends up more significant than the others, try eating the meal for lunch rather than dinner.

Don't Lay Flat If You Sleep

Lying flat presses, the contents of the stomach against the LES. Gravity helps to reduce the pressure with the head higher than the stomach. Position bricks, stones, or anything that's solid and stable under your legs at the head of your bed, using wedge-shaped pillows under your head and shoulders.

RECIPE#20 ASPARAGUS QUICHE

This fantastic tasting, balanced quiche fills you up with protein rather than fat!

Who doesn't like going out and ordering the balanced veggie quiche for breakfast? But who did know what you're eating is full of cream butter and cheese? That is a lot of milk and a lot of later regret. It tastes and looks like you're putting a lot of effort into it but it's straightforward.

We have done a couple of things that make this traditional recipe healthier. Turkey's bacon replaces standard bacon to cut down on fat. Swiss and Parmesan cheeses are used, full of flavor, which helps you to reduce the overall fat content of the recipe and still get the enjoyment of the cheese. BUT cream is the main culprit in this dish; half and half, the lowest fat cream, yet contains 18 percent fat! Replacing the cream with plain, non-fat yogurt creates the same creamy texture, but for your health, it is much better.

Ingredients:

unbaked,9-inch piecrust

1/2-pound asparagus cut into 1/4-inch pieces (or between 1 and 1 1/2 cups)

6 turkey bacon strips, cooked to the desired crispness and chopped

2 Tablespoon green onion or chives 3 eggs (or 2 eggs and 2 egg whites/ 1 egg and 3 egg whites)

1 1/2 C non-fat or low-fat plain yogurt (Greek yogurt can be used but can be more tart in flavor)

1/2 cup Swiss cheese

Directions:

1.   Preheat the oven to 4500, cover the piecrust with foil in aluminum, bake for 5 minutes, remove the foil and cook for 5 minutes.

2.   Steam asparagus to bright green and tender, yet crisp (about 4-5 minutes).

3.   When cooking the asparagus, in a bowl beat the eggs and slowly add 1/2 cup of yogurt at a time.

4.   Add salt, chives and whisk in the nutmeg.

5.   Add in the cheeses slowly, leaving a small amount to sprinkle over the quiche.

6.   When bacon has been fried, add the mixture to the egg.

7.   When the piecrust is finished while the asparagus is steamed, spread the asparagus across the piecrust's bottom.

8.   Pour the egg-yogurt mixture gradually over the top of the asparagus; this will give a layered look to the final product.

9.   Sprinkle over the quiche with remaining cheese.

10.   Reduce the temperature of the oven to 4000 and bake the quiche in 10 minutes, then reduce 3500 heat and start cooking for 25-30 minutes. The quiche is done by putting a knife in the middle of the quiche and coming out clean.

11.   Let stand before serving for 15–20 minutes. It means the quiche isn't going to fall apart.

Nutritional information: 200 calories, 11 g of fat, 16 g of carbohydrate, 2 g of fiber, 10 g of protein, 83 mg of cholesterol, 335 mg of sodium

2.2 Don't Have Too Much Alcohol

Alcohol increases the amount of acid released by the stomach and relaxes the lower esophageal sphincter (LES). If you want to have any drink during your celebrations,

Dilute alcoholic beverages with water or soda party. Limit consumption of all to one or two mixed drinks, to a maximum of 16 ounces of wine or three beers. Drink white wine rather than red wine. Choose the wine or non-alcoholic beer. Keep track of which alcoholic beverages make your heartburn worse, and avoid it as much as possible.

RECIPE#21 SIMPLE FERMENTED VEGETABLES [VEGAN]

Ingredients

1-2-pound organic carrots cut into sticks

1 bag of organic radishes, sliced

6-8 organic pickling cucumbers

1 quarter of filtered water

2-3 spoons of fine sea salt

2-3 sliced garlic cloves (or more)

A few sprigs of fresh dill

Directions

1.   Combine warm water and salt to prepare brine, and set aside to cool.

2.   Slice the garlic cloves and add as much fresh dill as you want to the bottles.

3.   To be slightly shorter than the pot, slice the radishes and cut carrots and pickles. Pack each one tightly into jars, as many as you can fit. Pour over the cooled brine and fill to the top to ensure the vegetables are completely covered.

4.   Twist over the cap and leave to ferment for 7-14 days at room temperature. Keep away from an area with fluctuations in heat like a stove. If you have any brine leftover, store it in the fridge and use it at a later point...6-8 Serves.

RECIPE#22 MATCHA GREEN TEA

Match, a traditional Japanese tea, is one of the most nutritious drinks you could eat. Bonus: This is also pretty yummy.

Ingredients:

- 1 tablespoon Match powder

- 6 ounces of hot water, break

Directions:

1. Boil 6 ounces of water.

2. Combine match powder and 1 ounce of hot water into a bowl.

3. Whisk quickly with a bamboo whisk, until the mixture forms a thin paste.

4. Apply more hot water to the paste mixture until it reaches desired consistency.

RECIPE#23 CHICKEN CUTLETS WITH SAUTE MUSHROOMS

In our house we eat lots of boneless, skinless chicken breasts. They're flexible, easy to prepare and a great lean protein source. In the freezer, we even keep a stash of cooked chicken breasts for quick and easy meals such as salads, stir-fries and tacos. This recipe includes white wine which may cause problems with GERD for some people. If you are one of them, just feel free to replace chicken broth.

P.S. —- The leftovers make excellent sandwiches. In the microwave, just heat the chicken and mushrooms, top with a slice of cheese and serve on a whole wheat bun.

Ingredients:

1 pound of boneless chicken breasts (or chicken breast cutlets) 1/3 cup of whole wheat flour

2 tablespoons of olive oil

3 tablespoons of butter

2 cups of mushrooms,

1/3 cup of sliced white wine (or low sodium chicken broth)

Salt and pepper to taste

Directions:

1.   Slice the chicken breasts in half cross-section, so you have thin chicken pieces, and trim any excess fat. (If you are using cutlets, skip this step.)

2.   The chicken is to be seasoned with salt and pepper.

3.   Place the flour in a tub, dredge the chicken in the flour until it is coated slightly.

4.   Heating the oil on medium heat in a pan.

5.   Add the chicken to the skillet, then brown on both sides for 3-4 minutes.

6.   Clear it from the pan when the chicken is cooked, and set it aside.

7.   Turn the heat to low. Add the mushrooms and butter to the same pan and sauté until the mushrooms are soft (about 5 minutes).

8.   When the mushrooms are finished add the broth of the wine or chicken to deglaze the pan and stir well.

9.   Returning the chicken to the pan and cooking it until the sauce has thickened (approx. 2 min).

Nutritional details (by serving): 289 calories, 9 g of carbohydrates, 18 g of fat, 26 g of protein, 329 mg of sodium Serves 4

2.3 Follow a Low-Carb Diet

It is no surprise there are a lot of useful definitions. There's a kale time and place, and a cupcake spot and a time. The advantages of complex carbohydrates and how to make sure you eat the right balance of carbohydrates, fat and protein. Discussing now the healthy eating guidelines:

Choose Whole Foods

We contain no such items as artificial sweeteners or fake meat. Lots of vegetables and legumes will be seen, such as black beans and lentils, nuts and seeds, such as almonds and chia seeds; and some healthy carbs, such as 100 percent whole-wheat flour.

I'll also teach you how to swap some of your favorite ingredients for more nutritious options (but still delicious). For example, standard pasta can be exchanged for whole-wheat pasta or vegetable noodles. Try avocado where you might typically be using mayonnaise. Ultimately, you might find yourself skipping bottled salad dressing, often loaded with heavily processed oils and sugars, and getting yourself made for a salad dressing.

A few ingredients might sound unfamiliar in the book, such as tempeh or nutritional yeast. (For the record, nutritional yeast is just deactivated yeast. It has a sweet, nutty taste that can be a great substitute if you avoid dairy. It's also a great source of protein.) Don't worry, though — most of these recipes will use ingredients that you already have in your kitchen.

Meal Planning and Prep

Meal planning needn't be complicated or time consuming. Thinking ahead about what meals you plan to make for the week can help you eat a healthier diet, save money in the grocery store, and avoid a one-ingredient last-minute trip to market. Even if you shoot for just one or two vegetarian meals each week, preparing a little will make a big difference. Preparing a few meals, or even just a few moves, will keep you on track ahead of time. Takeout is less enticing when dinner is already in the fridge. But don't worry, I won't be asking you to waste all of your Sunday lentils cooking. Just a couple of shortcuts can help speed you through the process. Here are a few tips for preparing meals:

Make a large batch of quinoa in a rice cooker or on top of the stove if you don't have a rice cooker. Quinoa can be used in lots of recipes, just like pasta. Cooking a batch ahead of time makes soups, stews, salads and wraps simple to add to a scoop. Clean and cut stuff like celery and carrots from the grocery store as soon as you get home. Such vegetables are often used as a foundation for soups and sauces, and are stored well in the refrigerator. Instead of buying precut fruits and vegetables that might be quite expensive, consider buying frozen produce that tends to be cheaper. Frozen vegetables in soups and stir-fry's are delicious, and do not require any washing or chopping. Frozen fruits can easily be thrown into a bowl of smoothie or yogurt without any extra preparation work.

Whisk a large batch of vegetables together. Sweet potatoes, broccoli, and green beans are especially great choices to roast in advance. I love to sprinkle roasted vegetables with salt and pepper and place them in my favorite salads, but they can easily be added to wraps, tacos and sandwiches as well. Don't buy food you're not going to be using. Many people are wasting money on food they think they should eat even if they don't like it. Do not load your cart with broccoli, if you hate broccoli. Choose a green vegetable you'll want to eat. Food in your crisper drawer which goes terrible won't do you any good.

BALANCE YOUR PLATE

You will notice that this cookbook contains a balance of carbohydrates, protein and fat in its recipes. Nutrient balance is essential, because while the carbs provide you with energy, protein and fat will help you feel relaxed and complete. Don't skimp stuff like avocados and olive oil on the healthy fats. Such components are essential to help your body feel full and satisfied.

Since vegetarian recipes typically don't have a significant source of protein, it can be difficult to formulate new diner ideas. This book will help you to rethink your plate and provide you with new ideas for good, fulfilling food. New dishes can be especially difficult for children, especially when the ingredients look unfamiliar. Whether it's Brussels sprouts or hummus when introducing a new element, it can sometimes help to pair it with something familiar. For example, pair it with baby carrots or cucumbers instead of serving hummus with an unknown vegetable.

EAT SENSIBLE PORTIONS

Not to forget the importance of correct portions. Even if you overeat, healthy foods aren't so good. All of these recipes have moderate portion sizes. To some people, eating smaller meals with more snacks in between could be better. Others may prefer 3 bigger meals.

If you do, make sure you don't eat until you're completely stuffed. Watch out for the hunger signals and eat slowly so your body has a chance to let you

know when it's enough. Many of these recipes contain foods that are "high-volume," meaning you can still have a substantial portion without over-eating.

RECIPE#24 BLACK BEAN BURGER

Black beans have protein and fiber, making them a very healthy addition to your diet. These are also an ideal low-calorie alternative to meat when you're in a "burger" mood. Tortilla chips and cilantro give this recipe a taste with southwestern twist enhanced by bacon, green pepper and a range of GERD-friendly seasonings. Be sure to pack them firmly together when forming the patties, and chill them in the refrigerator, so they do not fall apart when flipped. Also, meat eaters would find them so moist and tasty.

Ingredients:

2-15-ounce cans of black beans drained

2 eggs

1/3 cup of chopped green pepper

2 TBSP Flour

2 TBSP chopped cilantro

1/2 tsp ground cumin

1/2 tsp ground coriander

1/4 tsp salt

1/4 tsp Divided pineapple slices Iceberg lettuce 6 whole-wheat buns

1/2 cup baked tortilla chips, crushed

1/4 cup vegetable oil,

Directions:

1.   Lining a rimmed baking sheet with 3 layers of paper towels and spreading the drained beans over them.

2.   then Mash drained beans in a large bowl, add eggs, flour, seasonings, and crushed tortilla chips.

3.   Form into 6 patties, chill for 1 hour.

4.   In pan, heat 1 tbsp. oil. Place 3 burgers carefully in the skillet, and cook for 5 minutes.

5.   Flipping over and cooking for another 3 to 4 minutes until crisp.

6.   Removing and keeping it warm; repeat with 3 burgers leftover.

7.   Serve with GERD friendly condiments on whole wheat buns, and top with pineapple.

Nutritional details per serving: 360 calories, 1 g of sat fat, 697 mg of sodium Recipes 6

RECIPE#25 ASPARAGUS AND GREEN BEAN SALAD

Asparagus and green beans carry nutrients and are fantastic foods that promote good health and digestion. They are also full of flavor, tossed in this GERD sensitive recipe with a Dijon mustard vinaigrette. Certain ingredients include bacon, sausage, and shredded carrots giving your palate a savory mix. Preparing in advance is simple and delicious on a hot summer day. Enjoy it!

Ingredients:

1-pound fresh asparagus

1-pound French beans

2 TBSP shredded carrots

3 to 4 slices turkey bacon, cooked

3 hard-boiled eggs

2 TSP Dijon mustard

4 TSP balsamic vinegar

3 TBSP olive oil

Shredded salt and pepper

Directions:

1. Bring a large pot to a boil and add beans and asparagus, return to a simmer, then lower heat and cook until tender for about 4 minutes, do not overcook

2. Drain, rinse in cold water, and chill in refrigerator

3. Whisk the last four ingredients into the vinaigrette together, season to taste

4. Chop the cooled vegetables, add them to a salad bowl, and sprinkle with bacon and carrots.

5. Vinaigrette drizzle and egg top

Nutritional information per serving: (1/12th)–211 calories, 1 g sat fat, 295 mg sodium Recipe serves 12

Chapter 3: Making life Tasty

Gastronomic reflux (GERD), salivary gland infection, sinusitis, poor dental hygiene, or even certain drugs is a common symptom of loss of taste. Agues are the medical term for a complete loss of flavor. A partial taste loss is known as dyspepsia. Shape loss is due to a break in the flow of taste sensations in the brain or issue with the perception of these sensations by the brain. While taste problems are common, total taste loss is rare.

Heartburn or gastric reflux is a frequent cause of taste loss. Regurgitated stomach acid in the mouth contributes to a loss of typical taste and a taste that is characterized as acidic or metallic. Another common cause of taste loss is mouth or tongue infection. In the same way, poor dental hygiene causes bacterial growth in the mouth and a loss of taste. Some mouth or tongue disorders, such as mouth ulcers, cancer, and tobacco damage, can cause loss of flavor.

Radiotherapy and medicines like antibiotics and angiotensin-converting enzyme (ACE) inhibitors also can result in loss of taste. Goodness issues can take months or even years to solve. There may be permanent loss of feeling, mainly if the mouth is the object of direct radiation therapy.

Loss of mouth taste can be a symptom of a severe condition. Seek medical attention immediately if your loss of feeling in the mouth is chronic or affects you. When you experience failure of consciousness, including other severe symptoms such as difficulty breathing, high fever (more than 101 degrees Fahrenheit), extreme fatigue, changes of your vision, or difficulties concentrating, look for immediate medical attention (call 911).The following signs can be other symptoms, which may vary depending on the underlying disease, disorder, or condition. Specific body systems can also cause symptoms that often influence the sense of taste.

Taste loss can be linked to additional symptoms affecting the digestive system, such as:

Signs, the dentist wants to know:

Abdominal pain, Blowing, Cough, Heartburn, Indigestion

Salivary gland symptoms which may occur together with taste loss. Species loss -accompany a loss of taste related to gland disease. Seek immediate medical treatment (call 911) if the taste is lost along with any other severe symptoms, including:

Vision changes or speech changes

High fever (greater than 101 degrees Fahrenheit)

Dullness on one side of the body

Skill on one side of the inflammation and infection in the upper respiratory tract, sinuses, and the mouth

Dryness on one side of the body Symptoms can be caused by inflammatory conditions, viruses, or diseases that affect the taste buds of the tasteful tongue.

Gastro esophageal reflux disease (GERD), which could be damaged by gastric acid and bile, has a similar effect on the surface of the tongue. However, taste loss can be caused by conditions that affect certain parts of the body, such as the nervous system. The body receives not enough vitamin or nutrient that is essential for nerve function in certain nutrient deficiencies, contributing to nerve dysfunction or injury. The sense of taste may be lost in the case of nerves inside the tongue.

Common causes of taste loss

A variety of other disorders, including:

- Gastro esophageal reflux (GERD)
- Bowel or ascending infections
- bad oral hygiene
- Radiating medications
- Speck
- Infection with the salivary glands
- Sinus
- Jorgen syndrome (an autoimmune disease with dry mouth and eyes)
- Smoking

Another trigger

Brain tumor, Head injury, Oral Stroke stroke-like symptoms that can be a warning sign of a possible stroke. The doctor or licensed physician will ask you some questions related to your loss of taste

- How long did you have a loss of feeling?
- What drugs are you taking?
- What are your other symptoms?
- Are you smoking?

What are the possible taste loss complications?

As a result of serious diseases, the loss of taste may cause severe complications and permanent damage if treatment is not pursued. When diagnosed as an underlying cause, you and your health care provider designs are essential to follow the treatment plan explicitly designed to reduce the risk of potential complications, including

Dehydration, Excessive weight loss, Malnutrition, Paralysis, Spread cancer and Spread of infection.

RECIPE#26 BAKED CHICKEN PARMESAN

Total Time: 60 min Prep Time: 15 min Cook Time: 45 min Servings: 4

Nutrition Highlights (by serving)

Three hundred thirty-one calories 19 g fat 10 g carbs 29 g protein Love Chicken Parmesan yet hate the burning of your old recipe causes? For many people, the traditional recipe's spices and higher fat content will cause their heartburn. This heartburn-friendly Baked Chicken Parmesan version can be a safe alternative to an old favorite. it takes about 1 hour from start to finish.

Ingredients:

Four boneless, skinless chicken breasts 1/2 cup seasoned bread crumbs

Three tablespoons grated good quality Parmesan cheese Splash of

Italian seasoning

salt

Four teaspoons of olive oil

Directions:

1.   Heat oven to 375 F.

2.   Coat a baking dish with vegetable spray and cook gently.

3.   Combine 1/2 cup seasoned bread crumbs in a small bowl, three tablespoons grated Parmesan cheese of good quality (not the stuff in a can), a dash of Italian seasoning and a pinch of salt. Blend well.

4.   Place four boneless, skinless chicken breasts patted dry on a tray and brush with four teaspoons of olive oil.

5.   Dredge chicken breasts in the bread-crumb mixture on both sides. Move to a baking platter.

6.   Sprinkle over the chicken with any remaining breadcrumb mixture.

7.   Bake uncovered, or until finished, for 35 to 45 minutes.

More about Modern Parmesan Chicken

Chicken Parmesan sounds like a recipe straight out of Italy, right? Well, it originated in the United States, despite its name and ingredients — tomato sauce, mozzarella cheese, and Parmigiano-Reggiano cheese. Italian-American communities have developed recipes that resemble their home country's food. Then immigrants from Parma, Italy, came up with this dish of chicken. Parmigianino means "in the style of Parma." Today's definition of Parmesan-Sequa recipes means something breaded and fried, sauced, and cheesed. Given its state-of-the-art history, Parmesan chicken recipes are rooted in Italy. Consider your cousin Melanzana Ella Parmigianino or Eggplant Parmesan. It's a toss-up about where this dish originated.

RECIPE#27 FROZEN CAPPUCCINO GRANITA

Total Time: 10 min Prep Time: 10 min

Servings: 5 (3/4 cup each)

Nutrients: 73 calories 1 g fat 16 g carbs 1 g protein

A granite is a handmade frozen Italian dessert with a slushy texture. This dessert on a hot day is light and refreshing and will appeal to all of you coffee lovers there. Milk free from lactose makes it suitable for a diet.

Ingredients

2 cups of extra-strong brewed coffee

Five teaspoons of unsweetened cocoa powder 1/3 cup of sugar

1/8 teaspoon of ground cinnamon

1/2 teaspoon of vanilla extract

1/2 cup of lactose-free whole milk

Direction:

1.   Since flavors are muted when icy cold, use your preferred brewing method to make extra-strong coffee. Clear up a flat space in the freezer.

2.   The shelf at the rear and the bottom is coldest. Have a 9-inch round handle or 8x 8x2-inch pan, preferably ceramic. It can be used with glass or ceramic, but it will freeze even quicker.

3.   Put cocoa powder in a medium-sized bowl. While coffee is still scalding (reheat if yours has cooled), add about 1/4 cup of coffee to cocoa powder, and whisk to make a smooth, thick slurry slightly thicker than heavy cream.

4.   Add 1/2 more cup of coffee, and stir until mixed. Stir the remainder of the coffee back.

5.   Stir in sugar and shake until it dissolves. Whisk in sugar, cinnamon, and coffee.

6.   Pour into the baking pan and allow the mixture to refrigerate to room temperature. Remove the liquid, as the cocoa may have settled down, and place it flat in the freezer.

7.   The mixture will start freezing along the edges after 1 to 2 hours (the duration of this will vary based on your freezer temperature and the size of the pan). Use a fork to clear ice crystals from the sides of the pan and corners to the bottom, with the tines curving downward. Mix the rice and liquid to redistribute, breaking up the larger chunks. Continue scratching, cracking glass, and mix every 1 to 2 hours. The mixture turns slushy. Continue until no liquid left and frozen solid slush. When fully frozen, run the fork over the mixture and scrape again to produce thin flaky crystals (use some elbow grease!).

Ingredient

Variations and Replacements

Swap 1/4 teaspoon almond extract with coffee, or use a mix of both.

Cooking and Serving Tips

Adding chocolate to the hot liquid "blooms" cocoa; make it more nuanced and accessible in taste.

Serve in champagne or martini glasses with a dollop of whipped cream and a drop of shaved chocolate for a good show.

If you're sensitive to caffeine, use decaf coffee so you can enjoy an evening treat without staying awake! Instead, an afternoon pick-me-up of caffeinated coffee. In hot weather, ice bowls or glasses of wine for 20 to 30 minutes before serving to slow down the melt. Granite will keep frozen in an airtight container for several weeks. If required, re-flake the granite just before serving.

RECIPE#28 CHICKEN POT PIE RECIPE

Total Time: 55 min Prep Time: 15 min

Cook Time: 40 min Servings: 4

Nutrition Information (by a meal)

Four hundred thirty calories 12 g fat 49 g carbohydrates 34 g protein This chicken pot pie is made from heartburn-friendly ingredients comprising of skinless chicken breasts and skims milk.

Foods with high-fat content are usually the culprit that causes heartburn sufferers. This low-fat meal adds chicken pot pie to the table.

Ingredients:

1-pound boneless, skinless chicken breasts

1/2 teaspoon salt

One tablespoon of olive oil

1 cup of frozen carrots, thawed

drained 1 cup of frozen peas,

thawed and drained 1 (14.75-ounce) cream-style corn

3/4 cup skim milk, split into 1/4 cup and 1/2 cup portions

1 cup biscuit mix

Direction:

1.   Heat oven to 400 degrees Fact the breasts of chicken into 1-inch cubes, and season with 1/2 teaspoon salt.

2.   Heat 1 spoonful of olive oil or vegetable oil over medium to high heat in a skillet.

3.   Attach the 1-pound breast cubes of salted chicken and simmer for 8 minutes, stirring occasionally or until browned.

4.   In a 3-quarter baking dish, put the chicken and add 1 cup of frozen, thawed and drained carrots, 1 cup. Bake and cover for 25 minutes.

5.   Combine 1 cup biscuit mixture, and the remaining 1/2 cup skim milk into a mixing bowl. Remove until the dough forms soft.

6.   Clear from the oven and reveal a baking dish. Spoon dough with a tablespoon on chicken and vegetables, then spread evenly to cover the entire chicken mixture sheet.

7.   Bake until the biscuits are golden brown.

More Of Chicken Pot Pie

Chicken Pot Pie is at its highest a comfort food. It is the perfect vehicle for grilled or leftover roast chicken and vegetables combined with gravy or sauce. The crust is where one can get into trouble. High-fat pastry dough or puffed pastry crusts are typically used, which can cause heartburn sufferers problems. This is a lighter version of this Recipe.

Pot Pie History

Meat pot pies date back to the Roman Empire where they were served at sumptuous banquets, sometimes with live birds under the crust .The English gentry of the 16th century retained the tradition of meat pies made from bacon, lamb, game, and birds. This meat pie craze spread to the New World, which eventually took them to the West, where they became firmly entrenched in the culinary repertoire in the United States. Others claim the English pasties, favored by Cornish tin miners, are indeed a compact variant of a traditional pot pie. You have to say.

3.1 The Pros and Cons of Acid Reflux

The acid reflux diet is designed to help alleviate chronic acid reflux pain, known as gastro esophageal reflux disease (GERD). It is founded on the assumption that diet leads to painful symptoms, such as heartburn, regurgitation, throat pain, or heaviness. It may help to eliminate certain foods, especially spicy, tangy, or acidic ones.

After a process of temporary elimination, the diet plan can help you identify trigger foods. It's not a surefire way to remove symptoms, one but most of the time, if you find trigger foods; you might want to avoid them. Keep on reading to learn about the acid reflux diet's pros and cons and decide if it's right for you.

PROS

- Nutritionally well-rounded
- Not necessarily restrictive
- Non-cost-prohibitive
- Numerous recipes available

Generally safe for all populations, force you to give up some of your favorite foods

Doesn't work for anyone with acid reflux Maybe restrictive during the phase of elimination

The acid reflux diet, from cost to safety to longevity, proves itself to be a generally healthy diet that is suitable for most people. You shouldn't feel deprived of the acid reflux diet, because you will still be able to eat a variety of foods to keep you satisfied and avoid boredom. The acid reflux diet has no obvious nutrient deficiencies and contains all the prescribed food groups; the acid reflux diet is close to the Mediterranean diet in many respects. You should consume plenty of vegetables and leafy greens, whole grains, and low-fat proteins— and some research suggests that the Mediterranean diet may be as effective in treating GERD patients, the chronic form of acid reflux, as medication3.

Sustainability and Practicality

Because the acid reflux diet helps you to enjoy a variety of foods, long-term adherence shouldn't be difficult. The initial phase of elimination is only temporary, and even then, you won't find yourself skipping dinner parties with friends— as long as you make smart choices, this diet won't prevent you from eating at restaurants, office potlucks, family reunions, or other social activities.

Once you've recognized the causes, you'll definitely be able to suppress them to prevent symptoms.

Who The Diet Is For?

The acid reflux diet is tailored for a particular group of people: those with acid reflux. It is probably the most effective option to address the exact condition for that reason. Cutting off non-compliant foods like spicy foods and caffeine from your diet can help reduce or eliminate the uncomfortable side effects associated with acid reflux.

Cutting back on high-fat foods and refraining from eating large portions— two items, the acid reflux diet recommends — can contribute to weight loss. So, while the acid refluxes diet is not "intended" for weight loss, it can result in weight loss following it. Losing weight is the best way of reducing reflux symptoms for people who are overweight and who have reflux.

Energy and General Health

After spending some time on the acid reflux diet, you should notice that overall, you feel better. You may feel more energized, more inspired, and more productive; you may get better sleep and be in a better overall mood, and you may even feel stronger physically. That is because you are going to start fueling your body with nutrient-dense foods that optimize all the physiological processes of your body and help regulate hormones4.

Cost

This diet is not at all cost-prohibitive: you can make plenty of meals from any grocery store on an acid reflux diet. Indeed, the acid reflux diet could actually help save you money. Whether you tend to eat fast food or take-out a lot, the acid reflux diet would need healthier alternatives, so you can spare a few bucks by not driving through a drive-thru a couple of nights a week.

On the package, by buying frozen fruits and vegetables or sticking to those in season and on sale, you can save on the cost of the produce.

CONS

Overall, the acid reflux diet is suitable for most people, especially those with acid reflux who want symptoms to be minimized. Both foods, however, have disadvantages — the acid reflux diet is no exception. Here are a few inconveniences to remember before the acid reflux diet begins. As mentioned before, the menu for acid reflux is not meant to be restrictive, but there are always risks with any intake of elimination. You'll need to cut off foods that may intensify reflux symptoms, at least temporarily, so consulting with an expert is beneficial.

A physician or licensed dietitian will ensure that you maintain a balance and satisfaction of foods, without any feelings of privation.

Sustainability and Practicality

Again, the acid reflux diet will allow you to eat a lot of different foods, making it easy to adhere to in the long run. However, in the beginning, you may find yourself missing some of your favorite foods.

For example, if you usually eat pizza several days a week and cut it out because it's high-fat and contains tomato sauce for the acid reflux diet, you can feel disheartened when you can't eat pizza at a ball game, party, or another event.

Who The Diet Is For?

The acid reflux diet is intended for a specific population. Although it is usually nutritious and healthy for everyone if you have other objectives, this diet might not work for you.

The acid reflux diet is not necessarily meant to lose weight some other diet chart shall be maintained to lose weight.

Energy and General Health

Once you're used to a new healthy eating pattern, you'll probably feel better than ever before. You can find yourself moody and annoyed at the start though. But the benefit will outweigh the costs and the cravings will subside after a limited number of times. Try to concentrate on the food you can get and not on the menu you try to avoid.

Cost

Overall, the acid reflux diet is not expensive but some recommended foods may be costly. The menu, for example, emphasizes lean meat cuts which are often more costly than their higher-fat counterparts. You will also need to purchase lots of fruits and vegetables, which may seem expensive if you're used to eating low-cost processed foods such as cereal sugar or chips and salsa.

Although the acid reflux diet is generally safe for all populations, it is always best to consult doctor or dietitian before using a new diet plan. They'll be able to give you the best advice on whether your acid reflux diet is right for you.

RECIPE#29 LEMON CHIVE SALAD DRESSING

This is an easy and yet chic green salad vinaigrette. Using lettuce center Romaine, Boston or Bopp. Prepare this seasoning and about an hour before eating, in order to thoroughly add the chive flavor. Mind to toss before serving well. The downside here is that you use lemon juice, rather than vinegar. I consider the lemon juice is alkaline upon ingestion.

Ingredients:

Sea salt (pinch)

 1 lemon juiced

3 tbsp.;

6 Tbsp. extra fine sugar.

6 Tbsp. extra virgin olive oil.

Freshly ground black pepper

Directions:

1.   Mix the lemon juice, salt and sugar in the mixing bowl.

2.   Whisk until the dissolve sugar and salt.

3.   Start to whisk in the olive oil, chives and several pepper grinds.

4.   Keep whisking until it emulsifies dressing.

(Note: This dressing can be made for two by lowering the lemon juice to two tbsp. and the other ingredients by 1/3.) Keep leftover in the fridge container for potential use. It'll last for about a week.

RECIPE#30 CHICKEN AND RED POTATOES

it is a GERD-friendly recipe and a safe all-in-one meal overall. Extra-this delicious red potato chicken and crispy snack are perfect for company and versatile enough for busy school nights as well. Serve side by side with asparagus and a tossed salad or brown rice and you'll have a perfect, friendly meal. Enjoy it! Which makes Chicken and Red Potatoes an ideal meal for those suffering from GERD? Much of a potato's nutritional value lies in its skin. The thin, nutrient-filled coats, which are loaded with fiber, B vitamins, iron and potassium, make red potatoes exceptionally nutritious. The skin is already super light came, so the taste or texture does not detract from it. Chicken is an excellent source of protein, similar to harder red meat, while being comparatively more comfortable to digest. A great flower, rosemary is used to relieve heartburn while this recipe also adds a punch of flavor. Apple cider vinegar can give bowel protection to avoid acid reflux. The vinegar lowers pH levels in the blood to help the bowel system fight harmful bacteria and fungi.

Prep Time 15 minutes

Cook Time 40 minutes

Ingredients:

Approximately 300 g Red potatoes Cut into 1-inch cubes 2 large carrots peeled and sliced 1 tbsp. Grass-Fed butter

Directions:

1.   Preheat the oven until 425.

2.   Toss potatoes and carrots with the sugar, salt and turmeric mixed together. Spread evenly onto a baking sheet with rims. Squeeze the juice from the limes, and then apply to the baking sheet. Bake for about 35 minutes, stirring once midway, until vegetables are tender.

3.   Stir in rice, rosemary, olives and apple cider vinegar, move the roasted red potatoes and carrots to a casserole dish.

4.   Cook for another 15 minutes, until warm.

5.   Parsley garnishes, and serve hot.

RECIPE#31 SAVORY LENTILS WITH TEXMATI BROWN RICE

Ingredients:

1 lb. of organic lentils (2 Â1⁄2 cups), rinsed

8 cups of water or stock

1 onion,

3 garlic cloves chopped

2 carrots chopped sliced

2 stalks of celery

one bay leaf chopped

1⁄2 tsp dried thyme

Directions:

1.   in a pot boil water and lentils. Add materials.

2.   Reduce, partially covered, to the boil.

3.   Cook until tender (approx. 20 to 30 minutes), stir occasionally and add more liquid if necessary.

4.   Add sprigs of bay leaf and thyme. Season with salt and black pepper, freshly ground to match.

5.   Serve with brown rice over organic Teammate. Top with chopped parsley garnish. Serve with a light green salad, served in the above lemon-chive dressing.

3.2 Light Food Healthier Life

Proper gastro esophageal reflux disease (GERD) treatment often starts with a visit to a healthcare professional to get an accurate diagnosis. Recognizing that chronic reflux is not getting better on its own is critical. Over - the counter medications can provide short-term relief of the symptoms but can mask an underlying disease if it is used for a long time.

GERD treatment may include medicines recommended by your doctor and specific changes in diet and lifestyle. It may require a variety of methods, and some trial and error.

Changes in diets and lifestyles always start with what to avoid. These include factors that can cause symptoms or exacerbate them.

Coming with the right changes in diet and lifestyle involves finding out what works best for you. Not every cause and procedure will have the same effect on all people. Keep in mind that food can be just as important as what you're consuming. A particular food that induces reflux may be harmless earlier in the day when consumed 3–4 hours before bedtime.

GERD eating right doesn't have to mean cutting out all your favorite foods. Only making a few simple changes to your current diet is often enough. While there is no established "GERD diet," the following foods can help ease the symptoms or prevent them.

Fresh fruits: avoiding citrus fruits and juices such as oranges and lemons choose among other things from a number of non-citrus fruits such as bananas, melons, apples, and pears.

Livestock: Choose from a wide array of vegetables. Elite or May sauces or toppings high in fat or other irritants, such as tomatoes or onions.

Eggs: These are incredibly protein-rich. Nonetheless, if you're having an issue with eggs, stick to the whites and stay clear of the higher fat yolks that are more likely to cause symptoms.

Lean carnivores: High-fat meals tend to lower the pressure of the esophageal sphincter prolonging the emptiness of the stomach, increasing chances of reflux. Choose the grilled, poached, broiled, or baked lean meats.

Oatmeal, whole grain bread, couscous, and rice. All these are good sources of complex carbs that are healthy. Whole grains and brown rice enrich your diet with nutrition.

Certain root vegetables and potatoes: These are excellent sources of digestible fiber; however, as these are common irritants avoid adding onion and garlic during the preparation.

Fat is a nutrient category–high in calories but an essential part of your diet. Not every fat is created equal. Generally, avoid or reduce saturated fats and Trans fats (in processed foods, portions of margarine, and shortening). Try to replace them with unsaturated plant or fish fats in moderation. Types are Monounsaturated fats. Examples include oils like olive, sesame, canola, and sunflower; avocados; peanuts and peanut butter; and various nuts and seeds.

Fats that is polyunsaturated. Examples include oils such as safflower, soy, corn, flaxseed, and walnut; soybeans and tofu; and fatty fish such as salmon and trout.

Other Good Tips

Gum chew. Chewing gum (not spearmint or peppermint that can relax the LES) increases the production of saliva and reduces the amount of acid present in the esophagus.

Evicting alcohol. Alcohol is a known irritant, which can weaken the symptoms of LES and cause reflux. While some people may experience symptom spikes after just one drink, others may tolerate moderate amounts. Experiment seeing what would best for you.

Keep good posture on and off the meal. Sitting up when feeding is a good idea and stop lying flat for at least two hours after eating a meal. After a meal, getting up and walking around helps encourage the flow of gastric juices in the right direction.

Avoid eating straight away before bed. The amount of gastric acid contained in the stomach is increased by digestion. As you lay down, the LES ability to prevent stomach contents from traveling up the esophagus is weakening. Timing can differ from individual to individual, but in general it is not advisable for GERD sufferers to eat a full meal less than three or four hours before bed.

GERD eating healthy doesn't have to mean leaving out all your favorite foods. The aim is to build a diet based on a wide variety of foods including fruits and vegetables, lean protein sources, complex carbohydrates and healthy fats.

When you think foods can cause or exacerbate your GERD symptoms, try to keep a regular one-week diary.

A hot chest burn, a bitter taste in the mouth, a gassy stomach bloating –acid reflux is no picnic. Nonetheless, whatever you eat can have an effect. The best and worst acid reflux foods could spell out the difference between sweet relief and sour misery.

What makes Acid reflux worse?

Acid reflux happens when the sphincter at the base of the esophagus is not functioning correctly, causing the acid to reach the throat from the stomach. The worst reflux foods can worsen unpleasant symptoms, while other foods can soothe them, says gastrointestinal surgeon. Dietary changes significantly affect acid reflux.

Best Acid Reflux Foods

Best vegetable, protein, and fruit-balanced diets. Some of the best acid reflux foods include:

Chicken breast-make sure the fatty skin is removed. Skip fried, and pick baked, broiled or grilled instead.

Lettuce, celery, and sweet peppers–these light green vegetables are gentle on the stomach–and will not cause painful gases.

Brown rice–this carbohydrate complex is mild and satisfying–just doesn't fry it.

Melons-Watermelon, cantaloupe and honeydew are all low-acid fruits among the best acid reflux foods.

Oatmeal–Filling, hearty and healthy, this comfortable standard breakfast also works for lunch.

Fennel–This crunchy low-acid vegetable has a mild licorice taste, and a natural calming effect.

Ginger–Steep caffeine-free ginger tea or chew for a natural tummy tamer on dried low-sugar ginger.

Worst Foods for Reflux

In general, you should avoid anything that is fatty, acidic or highly caffeinated. The worst foods on the list of acid reflux include:

Coffee and tea–caffeinated drinks worsen acid reflux. Look for teas that are free of caffeine.

Carbonated drinks–Bubbles spread in your stomach, creating more pressure and more pain. Use plain water, or iced tea free of caffeine.

Chocolate-This treat has a trifecta of problems with acid reflux:

caffeine, fat and cocoa.

Peppermint-Don't be fooled by its reputation for calming the tummy; peppermint is the trigger for acid reflux.

Grapefruit and orange-The high acidity of citrus fruit relaxes the sphincter of the esophagus and worsens the symptoms.

Tomatoes –Also avoid marinara sauce, ketchup and tomato soup- they are all high in acid naturally.

Alcohol-This has a double whammy effect: alcohol relaxes the sphincter valve immediately but also increases the development of stomach acids.

Fried foods–these are among the worst reflux products. Skip the French fries, the rings of onions and the fried chicken — cook at home on the grill or in the oven.

Late-night snacks–Avoid eating anything within two hours of going to bed. You can also try eating 4 to 5 smaller meals throughout the day, instead of 2 to 3 big meals.

It's good to speak with your doctor if your symptoms are not eased by the best foods for acid reflux. Other alternatives may include changes in lifestyle, medicines that can block the esophagus sphincter from the acid and surgical procedures.

If you have severe or frequent heartburn or acid reflux, it is essential to get a doctor's appointment. Chronic acid reflux leads to cancer of the esophagus.

RECIPE#32 PISTACHIO CRUSTED SALMON

Total Time: 60 min Prep Time: 15 min Cook Time: 45 min

Servings: 4 (3 oz. salmon and 3/4 cup mash)

Nutrition Highlights (per serving)

393 calories 18 g fat 33 g carbs 25 g protein

Salmon is one of the staple foods in a Mediterranean diet and is an excellent source of fatty acids in the omega-3. Such fatty acids are called polyunsaturated, and can help protect the heart by reducing blood clot risk, plaque formation, blood pressure, serum triglycerides and inflammation. Aim at eating fatty fish such as salmon, sardines, trout or mackerel at least once or twice a week to reap health benefits from these heartbeats.

The "crust" on the fish is made of pistachios containing protein, unsaturated fats and fiber, not to mention a beautiful green hue! Fresh lemon juice is a source of vitamin C and adds a bright flavor so you don't have to douse your salt food. Serve the fish with a comforting side of potatoes mashed with celery root.

Ingredients:

1 big celery root, peeled and diced (about 3 cups diced)

3 medium yellow or white potatoes(about 3 cups diced)

2 tablespoons unsalted butter

1/2 cup low-fat milk

1/2 teaspoon salt and black pepper

12 ounces salmon

1 tablespoon Dijon mustard

1/2 medium lemon juiced

Directions:

1.   To make the potato celery root mash: place the diced root of celery and potato in a large pot. Bring to a boil and cover with water. Simmer for 20 to 25 minutes, until the source of celery and potatoes are soft. Drain, and go back to the bath.

2.   Add the butter, milk and salt to the root of the celery and the potatoes, and mash until smooth.

3.   Fish to make: Preheat the oven to 375F. Blot the fish dry and put the skin side underside down on a foil or parchment-lined baking sheet.

4.   In a cup, combine the mustard and lemon juice together and pour over the salmon until spread evenly.

5.   Pulse the pistachios until they look like breadcrumbs. Pulse the garlic, breadcrumbs, and olive oil until mixed.

6.   Spoon the fish with the pistachio mixture on top. Bake until the fish is cooked and flakes easily with a fork.

7.   Garnish with fresh chopped parsley, the celery root potato mash and salmon.

Ingredient Variations and substitutes

plant foods give omega-3 fatty acids such as walnuts, soy foods, chia seeds and soil flaxseeds. Try this recipe with drained and pressed tofu instead of salmon for a vegetarian-friendly dinner. Cut the tofu into thick slices and spread overtopping with lemon-mustard and pistachio breadcrumb. Note that tofu's3-ounce serving contains 80 calories, 4 grams of total fat, and 8 grams of protein, while salmon's3-ounce serving contains twice that number.

Cooking and Serving Tips

Celery root is a vegetable that tastes like a cross between a celery stalk and a turnip. It is a bulbous, thick peeling root. Trim the ends off and peel with a vegetable peeler to prepare the celery root, then slice or dice and cook.

Celery root brings to mashed potatoes freshness and lightness that preserves the warmth of the dish but also prevents from feeling too sluggish. One cup of diced celery root contains less than 80 calories and about 3 grams of fiber.

RECIPE#33 CHICKEN NOODLE SOUP

This Heartburn-friendly Chicken Noodle Soup with Vegetables is a good meal in a pot. Once a no - no for patients suffering from heartburn and acid reflux, this low-fat version makes this classic feel-good food appealing to those with digestive problems.

Most chicken soups are iridescent, with golden chicken fat globules. Protein is a known cause for nausea with heartburn and acid reflux, so this meal made from freshly cooked boneless, skinless chicken breasts is a godsend.

If the chicken breasts are prepared in advance, this simple soup recipe can be ready in about 35 minutes, making it a perfect busy weekend dinner.

Ingredients:

1/2 teaspoon of olive oil

1 cup of cut and diced celery

2 quarts of tea

2 cups of peeled and chopped carrots

4 cubes of low sodium chicken bouillon 1/2 teaspoon of thyme 1/2 teaspoon of salt

3 ounces of uncooked egg noodles

2 cups of diced, cooked skinless chicken breasts

2 cups of frozen peas

Directions:

1.   Add 1/2 tablespoon of olive oil to a large saucepan. Add 2 cups of celery trimmed and diced, and sauté until translucent over a medium - high flame.

2.   Add 2 quarts of water, 2 cups of peeled and chopped carrots, and 4 cubes of low-fat bouillon chicken, 1/2 teaspoon thyme, and 1/2 teaspoon salt. Take to boil.

3.   To the boiling water apply 2 cups (3 ounces) of broad egg noodles. Reduce heat and cook for eight minutes or until tender noodles.

4.   Add 2 diced cups of boneless skinless breast chicken meat and 2 frozen peas. Reduce heat, cover and simmer for 5-10 minutes over medium-low heat.

Have a Stock of Cooked Chicken Breasts on Hand?

Cook a lot of boneless chicken breasts (using your favorite method of cooking— grilling, poaching, baking, sautéing, pan-frying, steaming, etc.) and then preserve them from having them on hand for cooked chicken recipes like this one. You can have a wonderful meal on the table in no time, as frozen chicken breasts thaw very quickly. Freezing whole cooked chicken breasts rather than diced chicken meat is a better idea. The latter would dry out quicker. Some recipes, as this one does, will call for cups of diced chicken, but others will refer to whole breasts, which are then diced. So, you can dice a few chicken breasts if you like, and leave some whole. Freeze for 3 to 4 months in a zip-top bag or other containers.

3.3 Enjoy Eat Travel

For many people, it may be a stressful experience to travel. For those suffering from gastro esophageal reflux disease (GERD), the normal annoyances-traffic, unpredictable roadwork, lengthy airport check-in and security queues, overbooked flights-are exacerbated by frequent heartburn discomfort and physical pain. If you've scheduled vacation time, these tips will help you stay heartburn-free while traveling.

Prevent food causes. While your holidays are in the planning stages, here are a few essential things to consider. Are you staying with friends or family? If so, let them know about your dietary restrictions ahead of time. Tell them that while they don't have to go to the trouble of creating a completely different menu for you, you'd like to have a couple of recipes that will not cause your GERD symptoms to flare up. You can also offer help in preparing food-then all of you can sit down to a meal that everyone can enjoy. Traveling can lead to symptoms of heartburn for a number of reasons, which can turn out to be quite the dampener on the trip you've planned. The change in habit can create anxiety that causes symptoms to worsen and many patients find this an issue. Staying seated for long periods can also increase the likelihood of symptoms, particularly after eating. If you experience symptoms at flying regularly, it is best to plan ahead and pack the appropriate medication to avoid symptoms. Most treatments work to prevent signs of heartburn from arising, as opposed to treating the symptoms, which can help the jet-setting sufferer from heartburn.

Here are ways for a heartburn-free summer to beat the painful symptoms:

Keep your weight down. Carrying extra weight along while traveling will

increases the pressure on the valve between the food pipe and the stomach, allowing the acid to escape from the stomach, causing symptoms to develop. Having said that, some abdominal exercises, such as stomach crunches can force acid out of the stomach, which can also cause heartburn. Waiting two hours after a meal before doing the exercise is best.

Sleep smart Heartburn can have a real impact on the quality of life, especially when it's frequent. Because when you are lying down, fluid from the stomach doesn't have to move upwards towards gravity, heartburn is almost always worse at night. It can have a real impact on sleep quality and a knock-on effect on how well you work the next day.

Raise the head of your bed with some books or blocks by about 6 inches (15 cm). Sometimes, you should try a pillow wedge. It's also found that lying on your left side decreases acid reflux. Sleeping on the right side seems to cause sphincter relaxation (the tight muscle ring linking the stomach and food pipe) that usually protects against reflux.

Plan ahead when you experience symptoms frequently while driving, it is best to plan ahead and pack the correct medication to prevent symptoms. Ask your pharmacist about options that prevent symptoms as opposed to treating them, which could benefit the sufferer from jet-setting heartburn.

Similarly, music festivals give frequent heartburn sufferers a lot of trouble; from lack of food choice to lack of sleep, be sure to plan ahead if you're going to one this summer. Propping up your head while you're sleeping will alleviate acid reflux discomfort, so make sure enough pillows are packed.

Know your triggers. Some foods can cause heartburn, with the typical culprits being spicy, acidic, rich and fatty foods. Eating sizeable meal-or eating late at night-can sometimes cause heartburn, or make it worse.

Overeating, or too soon, may also increase heartburn so take your time to eat and enjoy meals. Feeling stressed or rushed while eating can also cause more stomach acids to accumulate in the stomach. Overeating can worsen heartburn so if possible, opt for smaller portions.

Target the problem before symptoms strike a proton pump inhibitor (PPI) may help if you are a frequent heartburn sufferer and want sustained relief. By preventing the production of acid in the stomach, it prevents heartburn at the source. Its long-lasting effect means it can provide symptom relief throughout the day and night.

Ready to make sleep arrangements. This is also the time for inquiring about your sleep arrangements. Ask your friends or family, if you can raise your bed head once you get there. If you are in a situation where your needs can not be met, the foam or inflatable sleeping wedges are lightweight and can be found online or in medical supply stores for under $100.

Pack in Your Trip. If you have GERD, the following travel steps will be taken:

Select comfortable clothes. Make sure you pick loose-fitting outfits when it comes to packaging for your trip. Set one aside, too, for your travel day - it will make sitting a bit more tolerable for any length. For these occasions, sundresses and tunics (for women) and pants with elastic waists are ideal because a too-tight waistband can uncomfortably squeeze your stomach and cause stomach acid to back up.

Take medication for your heartburn. Take extra heartburn medication when packing your toiletries, such as Tums or Pepcid AC, if it's something you're using to treat your GERD symptoms. Make sure to keep a few in your carry-on bag if your luggage doesn't hit your final destination. If you are traveling to another country, it's particularly vital that you pack enough medication for your entire trip. It is hard to find prevalent medication in another country when you have several language and communication barriers in another country.

Hit the road. Here are a few more smart travels ideas for GERD people:

Plan ahead. Set the time of departure beforehand. Allow enough time to get on the road or get to the airport, without feeling hurried through screening. You will reduce your chances of getting heartburn by reducing the need for a hurry-a common source of stress. Grab some tasty snacks. You know best what foods will cause your heartburn, so take along for your car ride or flight small portions of healthy snacks. This will avoid the temptations of fast food rest-stops or snacks on-flight. (Of course, airplane fare is not known to be very enticing, but by saying, "No thanks, I'll pass," you will stop eating something just because it's given to you when the cart comes along.)Give yourself a break. Whether you fly or drive, you'll need to wear a seatbelt. Ironically, having one pulled over your abdomen can exacerbate GERD, just as a tight waistband can do. That is why taking lots of breaks are essential. Remember to stop in the rest areas along the way or stand up during your flight and take a stroll down the aisle.

Eating Out on Holiday. Once you've reached your destination, it's essential to manage your meal to avoid aggravating your GERD carefully. Stick with the GERD diet. Whether family gatherings, get-togethers at fancy restaurants, corporate dinners or cruise-line smorgasbords, meals frequently play a significant role during holidays. Once you reach your destination take the same precautions as you take at home. That means avoiding the "evil" things that can make GERD worse— such as fried, greasy, and spicy foods, such as alcohol, caffeine, and acidic fruits. Also, it means not getting too close to a bed time-the absolute minimum is two to three hours in advance. Get suggestions which are GERD compliant. If you're at a restaurant, let your server know about your dietary needs and ask for menu suggestions. Note that small portions are necessary for reducing heartburn and that entrances to the restaurant can be twice as large as the servings you eat at home. Request an appetizer instead of the main course if you don't have the ability to avoid eating everything on your plate. And ask your server at the beginning of the meal to put half of your entrée in a to-go bag. Be solid. Sometimes well-meaning friends and family members, even when they want to be supportive, can be your downfall. Don't let yourself be tempted to try "just a taste" or get a second aid if you know you'll pay the price later on. Remember-and your loved ones-that if you're coping with a bout of heartburn you won't be able to enjoy their company then. It is tough to avoid the temptations of overindulgence when they seem to be everywhere. However, as someone with GERD you are well aware of the possible implications. You know that if you take the steps that will save you from heartburn, you will be able to enjoy your holidays better. Keep your sleeping quarters as comfortable as possible, keep your travel time enjoyable and stress-free, and watch what you eat, when and how much.

RECIPE#34 BANANA PEANUT BUTTER SMOOTHIE

Low-FODMAP smoothies may present a challenge. Smoothies often rely on a lot of fruit to make them thick so FODMAPs can be very high. This winning mix of bananas and peanut butter makes use of a few tricks to produce a creamy smoothie that is as yummy as dessert as it can move.

Frozen fruit and ground chia seeds are two critical ingredients in making thicker smoothies. Prepare the frozen bananas in advance to have smoothies on hand. Peel the banana, split it into 6 pieces and store them in an airtight

container or zip-top bag in the freezer. Grinding chia seeds increases their thickening capacity in the first step of this recipe, plus you'll get some plant-based omega-3s.

Ingredients

- 2 teaspoons of chia seeds
- 1 cup of lactose-free yogurt
- 1 peeled, frozen banana
- 2 tablespoons of peanut butter
- 1/4 teaspoon of vanilla extract

Directions:

1.   In a dry blender, add chia seeds (do not add to the wet blender or stick to sides) and process into a powder for about 30 seconds. Turn off mixer. Chia seed powder may adhere to the blender's cover and sides; tap the sides or scrape them down with a spatula to collect them at the bottom.

2.   Remove cereal, peanut butter, frozen banana slices, and vanilla. Mix for 60 seconds. Stop and scrape down the blender, and move any chunks that have not mixed. Cover and pump blender again, for 30 to 45 seconds, until smooth.

Ingredient Variations and Replacements

One cup of lactose-free kefir may be used instead of one cup of lactose-free yogurt. Smoothie will be slightly harder than yogurt.

Cooking and Serving Tips

This recipe yields 2 servings; it is difficult to make less in a full-size blender. Share or refrigerate half of it with someone to eat later that day, or for up to 2 days. This smoothie will remain thick so it's a great breakfast or snack to make-ahead.

If needed add a few drops of stevia extract for a splash of extra sweetness. If you don't have a frozen banana before serving you can still make a thick smoothie by chilling it for 10 to 15 minutes.

RECIPE#35 SWEET POTATO TOAST WITH GINGER-HONEY ALMOND BUTTER AND KIWI

Nutrition Highlights (by serving): 277 calories 14 g fat 35 g carbs 8 g protein

don't think toasters are just for bread. Get ready to make your dream breakfast yourself. This "toast" recipe is a nutritious way to serve sweet potatoes and it is soft and flavorful, with several anti-inflammatory ingredients, plus no processed meal. Sweet potatoes provide a good source of nutrients such as vitamin C and manganese, plus filling fiber. They are also an excellent source of antioxidants-the anti-inflammatory properties of the phytonutrients in sweet potatoes have been shown. That's more benefits than you would get a piece of bread. We also add fiber-rich kiwifruit and flavorful heart-healthy almond butter to top this toast off. Bonus added: you can whip up the whole recipe in less than 15 minutes.

Ingredients:

- 1 medium sweet potato, peeled or unpeeled

- 3 table spoons almond butter

- 1/2 teaspoon almond honey

- 1/4 teaspoon almond ginger

- 2 medium kiwis, peeled or unpeeled

Directions:

1.   Slice the sweet potato into 1/4-inch slices lengthwise.

2.   Stir the almond butter, ginger, and honey together in a small bowl until mixed.

3.   At the high setting of the toaster, toast sweet potato slices until the sweet potato slices are soft and cooked through. Remember, you might need to toast 2 times or more to get them to this level.

4.   Spread the almond-ginger-honey mixture on one side of each slice of toasted sweet potato slices and top with kiwi slices.

The almond butter may be substituted for any form of nut or seed butter. Peanut or sunflower seed butter also works great and all have a calorie profile close to that. To give a protein boost, add a layer of plain Greek yogurt over the nut butter. Swap banana slices in for kiwi, for a potassium boost. If you have virtually fresh or frozen berries, use them for extra anti-inflammatory antioxidants instead of kiwi. Try pumpkin pie spice instead of ginger to further change the flavor profile. If you want to take this to-go breakfast, put the halves together like a sandwich, wrap them in foil and eat on - the-run. Pair for a balanced breakfast with a smooth chocolate match latte, or a third cup plain yogurt. You may need to run each slice of potato several times over a toasting cycle. Keep your toaster low-medium so that you can run it over multiple periods softening without burning it.

RECIPE#36 SWEET AND CRUNCHY FENNEL AND APPLE SALAD

Try this 5-ingredient lunch salad, weekend dinner or weekend brunch. For those who have heartburn, salad dressings are usually not a good idea, because all the acidity will wreak havoc on a sensitive stomach. Lightly dressed with olive oil, sweet apples, and fresh fennel, this salad is a great digestive aid. Rice vinegar seems to be best tolerated by many heartburn-prone folks and all that is required is a tiny splash.

Ingredients:

•   1 bulb fennel, thinly sliced

•   1 sweet apple (like delicious red), unpeeled and thinly sliced

•   2 table spoons of extra virgin olive oil

•   2 teaspoons of rice vinegar

•   1/4 teaspoon of kosher salt

Directions:

1.   In a medium bowl, put the fennel, apple, olive oil, and vinegar.

2.   Add salt to the ingredients, and then gently mix to blend.

3.   Serve at room temperature, or chilled.

If vinegar is troublesome for heartburn, you can leave it out very quickly and enjoy this salad dressing directly with the olive oil. As for the other star ingredient, use any form of seasonal apples for this salad and hold the peels on to get more fiber and antioxidants that protect the cells.

During the warmer months, fresh fennel can be found at most large chain groceries or on the farmers' markets. Select clean, unblemished, brightly colored, and scented bits. Take off the green stems and hard outer layers before slicing thinly. Use a mandolin for perfectly sliced fennel and apples; small handheld models are affordable and very user friendly.

Make this salad ahead, and store up to 24 hours in the fridge. Until serving, garnish the fennel bulb with a few of the bright green feathery "fronds." They are as stunning as they are flavorful.

RECIPE#37 HEALTHY SALMON SALAD WITH CELERY

Total Time: 5 min Prep Time: 5 min Cook Time: 0 min Servings: 4

Nutrition Highlights (per serving)

169 calories 9 g fat carbs 19 g protein

Are you sick of tuna salad? Whether in a sandwich or a scoop over a salad, after a while, tuna can become a bit boring. Try the salmon the next time you're looking for a fish salad! The fish not only looks very distinctive but also has many nutritional benefits over tuna. This recipe calls for canned salmon, but if you prefer (or have leftover in the fridge) you can also use fresh, cooked salmon.

Another reason the salmon salad is better for you is that you don't need almost as much mayonnaise for salmon salad as tuna, because salmon are naturally oily. (This recipe requires light mayo to keep fat and calories even lower.) To optimize the health factor, serve this salad in a healthy bread sandwich such as flax meal bread or on top of a green salad or stuffed with tomatoes or avocados. It is delicious in a wrap of lettuce too.

Ingredients:

- 1 (16-ounce) salmon (drained)

- 1/4 cup (minced)

- 1 medium stalk celery (minced)

- 1/4 cup mayonnaise

- 1/3 cup sugar-free pickle relish (see notice below)

- Optional: 3 cups of fresh herbs (cut)

Directions:

1.   Place the salmon in a bowl and disintegrate with a fork.

2.   Add the remaining ingredients, and mix together gently.

Ingredient Notes and Additional Recipes

Salmon has more nutritional value than tuna — it has 3 times the omega-3 fat plus twice the vitamin E, 3 times the foliate and a full-day supply of vitamin D. Canned salmon is also a good source of calcium, with a4-ounce serving having about 250 milligrams of calcium (this is because canned salmon contain edible soft bones, which are very dense in nutrients and contain many minerals).

Mt. Olive, which may be available at your local store, is a good brand of sugar-free sweet pickle relish. But if you can't find sugar-free sweet taste, you can use a natural sweetener with dill pleasure or chopped dill pickle and sweeten — if you wish.

If you want chopped herbs, dill, chives, parsley and tarragon to be added all work well. Either use one type by yourself, or try a combination.

RECIPE#38 STRAWBERRY BASIL SPARKLER

Staying hydrated is an essential part of taking care of your blood pressure and your overall health. Drinking plenty of water is obviously the best way to maintain a healthy level of hydration, but plain water can get boring, well, sometimes.

It's easy to understand why people sometimes turn to sugary drinks and sodas rather than water, but sugary drinks are an empty source of calories that provide little nutrition and sometimes contain lots of sugar and even sodium — not the healthiest choice. Reach for sparkling water instead of soda. The bubbles make it somewhat more fun than plain water, and you can savor it with any fruit or herbs you like! Only make sure the diet labels are read. Some sparkling waters contain sodium, so look for versions that are sodium-free and unsweetened. Or at home, you can whip one up. One of my favorite combinations for jazzing up a drink is this strawberry basil sparkler. Fresh strawberries add natural sweetness while basil gives the berries a bit of an earthy flavor that balances that. When you want a little more fun and flavor without all the sugars and calories, it is a great drink to reach for.

Ingredients:

- Ice

- Four strawberries, sliced

- Six basil leaves, roughly sliced

- 12 ounces of sodium-free sparkling water

Directions:

1. Stir ice into a glass of highball.

2. Add sliced basil and Strawberries.

3. Stir and top with sparkling water. Enjoy it!

Use any kind of fruit or herbs you like, with mint or thyme, such as blueberries, blackberries, citrus fruit, or apples. After that, you can munch on them, so choose your favorite! If you prefer, you can also use plain water. Make sure your sparkling water is unflavored and free of sodium so that your final drink is nutritionally friendly.

RECIPE#39 PAPAYA YOGURT & WALNUT BOAT

When snacking, try combining a protein fruit or vegetable with a little healthy fat. A combination of carotenoid and papaya rich in antioxidants with Greek yogurt and walnuts rich in omega-3 makes for a winning pick-me-up hit. Using plain yogurt to minimize added sugars (chilled papaya and a cinnamon powder provide enough natural sweetness). Papayas contain a healthy dose of fiber and potassium for good cardiovascular health, vitamins A and C for rejuvenation of skin and mucosal cells, and foliate that contributes to cellular metabolism. Papayas also contain papain, an enzyme that helps break down the proteins. Papain is being researched as a way to help break down the proteins in our digestive tract for its role in digestion. Walnuts are the most studied nut for cancer prevention because they contain high levels of polyphenols and other compounds that may be safe. Add them to snacks and breakfasts and, like this herbed faro salad with pomegranate and feta, also savory dishes.

Ingredients:

1 medium papaya, half

1/2 cup plain fat or low-fat Greek yogurt 1/4 cup walnuts

1/4 cup ground cinnamon

Directions:

1.   Scoop the papaya seeds off.

2.   Fill every half of the papaya with half of the yogurt, walnut halves, and ground cinnamon powder.

3.   Eat with a spoon, and scoop out papaya flesh bites.

Papaya can have a dense texture and flavor which some people don't like. Seek to cool the papaya before eating to reduce some of the unwanted feeling. Or, before filling with yogurt, fry the exposed papaya flesh with a cut lime.

You can try this with a half or quartered melon, like a cantaloupe or honeydew, as well. Fruit has the same colored orange flesh as papaya so it contains carotenoids too. Honeydew is rich in vitamin C, potassium and vitamins B. Planning to pack up this to-go snack? For more comfortable travel, you can peel the papaya, chop it into cubes and pile the meal in a container. Entertaining Breakfast Company? Serve half of papayas and set up a table with various fillings and toppings (think yogurt, walnuts, coconut flakes, chia seeds, fresh or dried fruits) so that people can make their own boats and style them. Don't forget to take a snapshot of the lovely (and nutritious!) creations of all.

Chapter 4: Managing Your Meals and Trigger Foods

This regurgitation is usually long-term and can lead to painful symptoms in the upper abdomen, including heartburn and discomfort. The severity of the condition has often to do with diet and lifestyle. Around 20 percent of the American population is affected by gastro esophageal reflux disease (GERD). Evicting triggering foods and following other dietary tips can ease GERD symptoms. In this article, we are addressing the foods that people with GERD may want to exclude from their diet and the feeds they may profit from consuming. Americans continue to blast extra calories with sugary drinks like soda — which come with a lot of health hazards. Research, including a study published in the American Journal of Public Health in November 2013, has linked soda consumption to the risk of heart disease and diabetes, as well as rising obesity rates.

Findings from a study on journal Appetite in August 2011 suggested that drinking soda can trigger sweet cravings by dulling your sensitivity taste, sparking a vicious cycle of eating fresh foods and drinks.

Sugar is so concentrated and invisible in soda. When telling people that a 20-ounce (oz.) bottle of cola contains more than 16 teaspoons of sugar, they're shocked. Overdoing it on both sugar and calories is just so easy. "That entire sugar intake has damaging effects. A study published in Diabetologia in May 2015 found that swapping out only one sugary drink a day reduces the risk of diabetes by as much as 25 percent.

Diet soda fiends are not off the hook either: A study published in the Journal of the American Geriatrics Society in March 2015 found diet soda consumption to be directly related to abdominal obesity in adults over 65 years of age. The waist circumference increase among diet soda drinkers was three times that in nondrinkers.

"While you don't get the same number of calories or sugar from a diet soda as you would from a regular diet, the belief is that the body senses the sweet flavor with diet soda and craves the calories that would typically go with that flavor. "As a result, people end up' making up' for the missed calories in other foods they eat all day long." In Kennedy's view, other unhealthy lifestyle factors "often go hand in hand with frequent soda consumption, compounding the health effect of soda. Often they don't make the best food choices when someone is having a mixer either. "So, what are some better options? There are plenty of other healthy, nutritionally-value drinks that you can drink rather than soda. Nevertheless, it is still important to consider what is in your soda replacements. Replacing soda with fruit juices that are high in sugar or tea and coffee drinks that are loaded with added refined sugar is not much better for your health. But swapping out soda for low-sugar beverages, such as unsweetened iced coffee or tea, can reduce your intake of sugar while adding beneficial antioxidants to the diet. Low-fat milk is also a better option, containing vitamins and nutrients, including calcium, for example. Want inspiration? Start with these healthy, low-calorie thirst-quenchers, which will undoubtedly still satisfy your taste buds.

RECIPE#40 LOWERS FAT PESTO AND BUTTERNUT SQUASH PIZZA

Most people love pizza. If you're having heartburn, pizza might not love you back. Sometimes enjoying a slice between the cheese and acidic tomato sauce leads to uncomfortable symptoms later. Why not enjoy a pizza which is lower in fat and acid? This version of pesto and butternut squash features simple homemade dough, sweet and creamy butternut squash, as well as a DIY pesto less likely to cause heartburn.

Ingredients:

1 package of dry active yeast,1 teaspoon of sugar,1 cup of warm water, 1 1/2 cup of whole wheat pastry meal,1 1/2 cup of all-purpose flour

1 teaspoon salt, 2 tablespoons of extra virgin olive oil, split, 1 cup of butternut squash, diced, 1/2 tablespoon of oil, 1/4 teaspoon of salt, 3 tablespoons of pesto

Directions:

1.   In a bowl mix the yeast, sugar, and water; stir and allow to sit for 10 minutes. In mixer equipped with a dough hook, put the flours and salt in the bowl to prepare the dough.

2.   Add the mixture of yeast and one spoonful of olive oil. Run the machine on low until the ingredients are just mixed, then increase the medium speed until the dough in a giant ball has come together.

3.   Transfer the mixture to an oiled bowl (using the first spoon) and cover with a clean towel in the kitchen. Let it stand for an hour. Store half the dough in a safe bag for freezer use another time.

4.   Approximately halfway through the rising money, preheat the oven to 400F, and prepare a sheet pan lined with parchment paper. Place butternut squash and drizzle with oil on the sheet pan, and sprinkle with salt. Roast until tender, in the 400-degree oven. Prepare pesto now, if you haven't already done so use a rolling pin to position the raised dough on a slightly floured surface, and roll flat. Remove the sheet pan carefully from the oven and drizzle with olive oil (second spoon).

5.   Move the dough to the saucepan and press the dough gently to the bottom. Top with pesto, squash ready and sprinkle with cheese. Raise temperature on the oven to 450F.Bake for 16 minutes and turn the pan halfway through the cooking once.

6.   When cheese is bubbled and crust is removed from the oven in golden brown, allowing it to cool slightly before it is sliced into 8 large slices.

Use any other veggie you want instead of the butternut squash; other suggestions for the taste include broccoli, bell pepper, black olives, or spinach. Or just mix and match! Both vegetables offer unique nutritional benefits. For a balanced digestive system, make the dough with whole wheat pastry flour increases the amount of full grain fiber. While preparing the dough ahead, you can make the whole pizza up to eight hours in advance and then leave it to bake later. Add the toppings, loosely cover with plastic wrap and store in the refrigerator if it will be more than two hours before you need to cook it. Place in the fridge overnight to defrost the remaining frozen dough. Before using, put in to room temperature.

RECIPE#41 LOWERS ACID MANGO COLESLAW

Total Time: 20 min Prep Time: 20 min Cook Time: 0 min
Servings: 6 (1 cup each)

Nutrients: 64 calories 3 g fat 10 g carbs 1 g protein

Traditional coleslaw recipes are filled with ingredients that can make heartburn worse, including raw onions and high-fat creamy dressings. Although some vinegar-based dressing is lower in calories and fat, they can often be problematic due to the use of citrus and vinegar. Rice vinegar tends to be less acidic, so it can be a good option for those who are experiencing heartburn and craving this classic side dish. Mango adds natural sweetness and a tangy edge, which heartburn-prone folks also tolerate well. Consider this much healthier and veggie-filled side dishes a batch for your next bob in the backyard.

Ingredients:

- 1⁄4 cup of rice vinegar

- 1 cup of canola or avocado oil

- Two teaspoons of sugar

- 1⁄2 teaspoon seeds of celery

- 1⁄2 teaspoon of kosher salt

- 4 cups of green cabbage shredded

- 1 cup of grated carrots

- 1 cup of fresh mango

Directions:

1.   Whisk vinegar, olive oil, sugar, celery seed, and salt in a large bowl.

2.   Remove chives, onions, and mango.

3.   Toss all the ingredients in the dressing well to paint.

4.   Enable to sit for at least 10 minutes before serving or covering at room temperature and put in the refrigerator for up to 12 hours before serving.

5.   For another fun version of this recipe, substitute mango with bell pepper. It lowers the sweetness well but does increase the snap.

6.   Add chopped parsley, cilantro or your favorite chopped herbs for an extra pop of green color and fresh flavor.

7.   To save time in the grocery store section, search for bags of pre-washed and pre-shredded cabbage and carrots.

8.   Allowing the coleslaw to sit for about an hour helps the aromas to get married and the cabbage to wilt slightly. This recipe will save over 200 calories per serving as

compared to regular versions based on the mayoral crowd-pleaser served this recipe with pulled pork, fish tacos, burgers, or grilled sausage.

RECIPE#42 CUMIN-SPICED SHREDDED CHICKEN, BARLEY, AND VEGETABLE SOUP

Here's a heartburn-friendly soup that's less than 300 calories per serving but heartfelt enough that you're not even going to make it. For those experiencing heartburn, balanced, portion-controlled meals like this are important — the smaller portions prevent the abdominal pressure, which in turn prevents reflux. Plus, if you're trying to lose weight as a way of controlling the disease, the lean protein and filling fiber in this soup will help you feel full for hours and eat less overall.

Ingredients:

2 medium boneless chicken breast, 1 tablespoon cumin

1 teaspoon dried oregano

1/2 teaspoon salt, 1/2 cup barley

2 medium carrots, peeled and chopped

1 14-ounce cannellini or other white beans, rinsed

1 medium zucchini, spiraled , 1 cup kale, chopped

Directions:

1.   Boil 8 cups of water and add the breast, cumin, oregano, and salt for chicken. Boil, covered, until a fork can easily pierce the chicken breast–about 15 minutes. Remove the chicken when ready, strain the liquid and set aside for use as the base for soup.

2.   Add barley to the liquid which is strained. Bring to a boil, and cook for about 20 minutes, covered. Attach the carrots and beans and cook for another ten to fifteen minutes, until the carrots are tender.

3.   Meanwhile the chicken shreds. Using your hands or two forks you will tear this apart. Stir in the chicken, kale and zucchini. Simmer, and serve for another 5 minutes.

4.   One single serving of this soup provides 22 grams of protein, 9 grams of fiber, and 2 grams of fat only. The protein comes from both the beans and the chicken but most of the thread comes from the seeds. This is a flexible recipe — uses your favorite grain or any one you have at hand. All legumes are a delicious, heart-healthy choice of food and they're easy to incorporate into different dishes, whether they're soups, stews, salads or sides, so have fun!

5.   Similarly, this recipe would hold up well on multiple whole grains. Barley is widely used in soups but instead you can opt for wild rice or brown rice.

6.   Spiraling the zucchini adds body to the final dish, and makes it fun to present. You can use a vegetable peeler to make zucchini strips if you do not have a paralyzer then slice them into 4 or 5 to resemble spaghetti strands.

Alternatively, you can just chop the zucchini and add them in the same way that the zucchini noodles would.

4.1   Steps and Precautions

Except for bottled water, most bottled beverages — including fruit and vegetable juices and herbal teas are preserved with ascorbic acid as part of the "canning and bottling" process and can, therefore, have a low pH value — meaning they are acidic and potentially irritant. Although many enjoy mint tea as a digestive aid, mint may cause relaxation of the muscle valve between the stomach and esophagus, allowing acidic digestive juices to leak into the esophagus. For this reason, "Gripe Water," a pediatric remedy that often contains mint and other herbs, may not be suitable for acid reflux.

Last but not least, while diet and lifestyle changes may be beneficial for GERD, some people also need acid-reducing medicine, so check with your doctor if you're struggling with more than just occasional heartburn.

The trigger-food diet

Many foods can cause GERD symptoms. GERD is a digestive disorder, and nutrition can often affect the condition's symptoms. Changes in diet and lifestyle can go a long way towards the treatment of many GERD cases. Foods that may aggravate the symptoms of GERD or reflux esophagitis include meat, as it tends to be high in cholesterol and fatty acid oils and high-fat foods, which may cause the sphincter in the stomach to relax high amounts of salt-rich calcium foods, such as milk and cheese, which are sources of saturated fat.

The researchers found that children often developed GERD symptoms after drinking cow's milk. Continuing research is investigating whether this applies to adults, too. People who experience nausea or frequently bloating after eating dairy products that contain cow's milk may find that removing them from the diet will minimize these symptoms. The relationship between cholesterol and GERD was explored in a study published in Alimentary Pharmacology and Therapeutics. The results indicated that it was more likely for people who consumed more cholesterol and saturated fatty acids and a higher percentage of fat calories to develop GERD symptoms.

The trigger-food diet includes removing popular trigger-foods to alleviate symptoms, such as coffee and chocolate. Such approaches have little scientific support, and the results vary from individual to individual.

RECIPE#43 CIDER APPLE VINEGAR.

Ingredients:

- 2 tbsp. of apple cider vinegar
- 2 tbsp. of organic concord grape juice (not concentrate)
- one and a half tsp of freshly grated ginger
- 6 oz. of cold water

Directions:

1. Place all the ingredients in a tall glass and stir vigorously to mix.

2. Add ice if you wish. For best results, drink in the morning or before meals.

Additional food flare-ups

Additional foods typically cause GERD flare-ups, which doctors often recommend to avoid people with this condition. These include chocolate mint carbonated drinks with other acidic beverages such as orange juice, coffee caffeine acidic foods, including tomato sauce. There is a piece of clinical evidence that these foods are associated with GERD symptoms, but some people's anecdotal experiences with the condition suggest that these foods may worsen symptoms. However, food triggers may vary from person

to person. People with GERD should try to eliminate every type of food from their diet to see if their symptoms are getting better.

RECIPE#44 SKILLET PEANUT BUTTER CINNAMON SPICE COOKIE

This decadent yet low-carb cookie is the perfect treat for someone with diabetes. It is made with blood sugar lowering cinnamon. Mostly, it's excellent!

Ingredients:

•   One large egg

•   1 cup natural peanut butter

•   ½cup brown sugar

•   ¼ cup almond meal

•   1 teaspoon vanilla extract, cinnamon and baking soda

•   1 teaspoon

•   ¼ teaspoon salt and ground ginger

•   2 tablespoons peanuts

Direction:

1.   Oven preheats to 350 Feat the egg in a bowl until slightly rubbishy. To combine well, whisk in peanut butter,

brown sugar, almond meal, vanilla extract, baking soda, cinnamon, ginger and salt.

2.   Sprinkle lightly with a non-stick spray on an ovenproof skillet. Pour batter into the skillet, and spread with a spatula evenly. Sprinkle the top with a few peanuts if desired, and slightly press down.

3.   Place the cookie on a rack in the center of the oven until the edges are puffed. Let cool and serve for 10 minutes before cutting.

Nut Butters: Even in your pantry, this recipe looks bare; it's easy to adapt based on what you've got on hand.

And if you're in the unfortunate situation of running out of nut butter, you can make your own by mixing a rounded cup of nuts in the food processor with a spoonful of oil until it forms a creamy spread.

Sweeteners which has a richer taste than white sugar, even if you could substitute it in a pinch. Pure maple syrup or honey may also be used, but be sure to reduce the oven temperature by 25 degrees and cook it for a few minutes longer to prevent burning.

Nut-Free Variation: If anybody in your household is nut-free, you can still make this cookie — just substitute the almond meal in sesame oil. Made from sunflower seeds, this is perfect for those with allergies to tree nut.

Vegan Variation: For a vegan version, use the seed egg chia. Mix 1 tablespoon of chia seeds with 3 tablespoons of water and let it sit to gel in the other ingredients for about 10 minutes before mixing. This trick is a good one to recall when eggs run out next time. If you feel additionally decadent, load this cookie with lots of healthy add-ins. In the mood for chocolate? Swap the almond flour for 1/4 cup of cocoa powder, or mix in 1/2 bowl of chopped dark chocolate, rich in antioxidant polyphenols and flavanols.[1] Do you want anything fruity? Stir in some frozen berries. This recipe with dried, wild blueberries is particularly delicious. Make a new nutty cookie with various types of nuts and seeds including walnuts, sunflower seeds, and almonds. To make a granola flavored cookie, add a handful or two of dried fruit along with those nuts. This cookie is best when undercooked a little bit. When you take it out, the center might not look entirely done, but it will continue to cook as it cools. To prevent sticking, be sure to use a non-stick or well-seasoned cast-iron skillet.

4.2 Best Drinking Practices

How a person drinks beverage can worsen acid reflux or heartburn, too.

Some practical methods for reducing symptoms:

Stay hydrated throughout the day, and avoids drinking large amounts in one sitting.

Do not eat drinks late into the night.

Stay standing upright after having something to drink.

Chronic acid reflux inspires any number of lifestyle changes, and beverage choices may be one of them. Many "go-to" drinks such as coffee and sodas are likely to exacerbate heartburn and other symptoms of acid reflux, known as GERD in its chronic form. If you're used to soft drinks or some fruit juices when you're thirsty, consider switching to alternatives that may relieve symptoms.

Naturally Alkaline Artesian Water

If you were taking chemistry in high school, you might know that liquids may be acidic, alkaline or neutral. The pH level is a measure of just how

acidic or alkaline a solution is. Besides further irritating inflamed esophageal tissue on the touch, acid also stimulates pepsin, the stomach enzyme which primarily functions to break down protein, which in effect turns into acid. That makes things worse. Much of acid reflux management is to avoid acid itself.

A July 2012 research in the Annals of Otology, Rhinology & Laryngology found that consuming high alkaline water at pH 8.8 instantly neutralizes pepsin, the digestive acid enzyme when contact is reached with certain substances. It was also shown to be an acid buffer that avoids direct acid contact with the esophagus. Drinking plenty of water, particularly when you suffer from acid reflux, is essential for good health. There are, however, two qualifications: First, water should be drunk throughout the day in smaller amounts to avoid regurgitation, a common problem with acid reflux. Second, water should not be consumed with meals in quantities because it interferes with digestion and can cause food to expand, stimulating the production of acid. Waters are nowadays available, but many contain sugar or artificial sweeteners. A healthier option is natural flavoring: simply add slices of your favorite fruits and veggies— lemons, bananas, watermelon, cucumber, mint, or limes — to an ice-cold water bottle for a refreshing and pleasant drink. Another great option is to put chopped fruit, add water and freeze in an ice cube tray. For instant flavor and color, growing these colorful cubes of fruit in your beverage!

Go Natural

Green Tea studies suggest that it can help to reduce the risk of different types of cancer, heart disease, obesity, kidney stones and probably even cavities. Besides this, green tea is calorie-free (if you do not have milk or sugar) and naturally high in antioxidants. Green tea comes in many varieties. Drink it hot or iced, and a few drops of honey will do you well if you want a touch of sweetening. Switch from traditional tea or coffee to caffeine-free herbal teas might be a good idea when chronic acid reflux becomes a problem. Tea made from leaves of Camellia silences — including "black" and green tea — and coffee both contain caffeine and other substances that may aggravate reflux of acids. Herbal teas can do more than just offer a neutral alternative. Chamomile and licorice teas have properties that may help to soothe the symptoms of acid reflux.

RECIPE#45 STRAWBERRY GREEN TEA ICE CUBES

Throw them into beer, tea and juice bottles or cups, or blend in smoothies to provide flavor boosts and antioxidant inflammation.

Ingredients:

- 3 bags of green tea
- 2 cups of water
- 1 cup of honey
- 1 cup of thinly sliced strawberries

Directions:

1. Water heat up and tea brew.

2. While hot, mix in the honey and stir to combine.

3. Allow to cool for up to 24 hours at room temperature, or put them in the refrigerator (with the tea bags in the mixture).

4. Pour a mixture of cooled tea into ice cube tray.

5. Place the ice tray in freezer and allow for a 15-minute freeze.

6.   Once 15 minutes have gone by and the cubes have started freezing, add a few sliced strawberries gently to each hub.

7.   Return the tray to fridge, about 3 hours to freeze. Leave the ice cubes in dishes once frozen until they are ready to use or transfer to a safe freezer bag.

Mix cooled tea with sliced strawberries instead of freezing into cubes, and pour over ice for a refreshing and low-calorie beverage. Swap for this recipe in any of your favorite sorts of tea and fresh fruits. White tea and raspberries, chamomile and blueberries, or lemon-flavored black tea with thinly sliced oranges are other flavorful combinations. Big ice cubes are an ideal option for large pitchers, large bottles of water or drink distributors, while smaller trays work better if you serve drinks in individual glasses.

Add Juice to Seltzer

There's no need to buy sugar soda or costly vitamin-enhanced waters— which also contain calories — when you can combine 100% non-sugar juice with seltzer instead.

Granite juice and grape juice are antioxidant sources that can help protect your brain and blood vessels. Still, don't take juice overboard. It's a common misunderstanding that juice is right for you because it's made from fruit. Although it does have the nutritional benefits of lacking soda, it can also be high in sugar and calories.

Mixing one-part juice with three parts of seltzer to reduce your sugar intake. Citrus juices, such as orange and grapefruit— together with cranberry, strawberry, cherry, and pineapple juices— are very acidic and can best be avoided. Apple, peach, and pear juice are almost as acidic as orange juice. Many vegetables and their juices are alkaline and are less likely to cause problems, including cucumbers, lettuce, and cabbage. Yet everyone is different, and learning from trial and error is good.

RECIPE#46 MIXED BERRY ICE CUBES WITH SELTZER

The body comprises of about 60 percent water. Water is a building material for cell life. It regulates internal body temperature through sweat and breathing, helps to metabolize nutrients, helps to flush waste through urination, acts as a brain, spinal cord, and fetus shock absorber, forms saliva, and lubricates joints.

If you typically drink sugar-sweetened beverages such as juices or sodas, try swapping in a glass of water to wean yourself off slowly. Watching their sweet beverage intake is particularly important for people with diabetes, because they can increase blood sugar very quickly. Many people with kidney problems may also need to watch for their rich potassium (i.e. orange juice) and phosphorous (i.e. sodas) drinks intake.

The bubbles in seltzer water emit a fuzzy feeling without adding any sugar. We want to get you hooked on wine! It is one of the best drinks one can drink.

Ingredients:

1/4 cup of blueberries

1/4 cup of blackberries

1/4 cup of blackberries

tap water

Directions:

1.   Divide the berries into a tray of 16 cube ice cubes. Add tap water to cover and place until frozen in the freezer (the best way to do that a day ahead).

2.   Place the desired quantity of ice cubes in a glass to serve, and top with seltzer water.

Toss some fresh herbs or lemon zest with the berries for extra zing, before freezing into ice cubes. Add the ice cubes to a batch of iced tea during the hot summer season. To reduce freezer burning, pop them out of the tray once the ice cubes are frozen, and store them in an airtight container.

Dairy and Plant Milk

If someone's been to the supermarket they know that milk no longer simply means cow's milk. Unless you're lactose-intolerant or otherwise allergic, the alkaline cow's milk may be OK, but it can also cause allergies for some people. Nonetheless, goat's milk is preferred over cow's milk, as it is easier to digest. There may well be better choices, though. Not only are plant-based milk made from soy or almonds healthy, but when the final product has a chemical structure, this can help to neutralize acid that lingers in the esophagus.

4.3 Holistic Dietary Plans for GERD

Some foods could actively improve the symptoms of GERD.

Researchers had not fully understood GERD until recently and there was a lack of scientific evidence to suggest that changing the diet might improve symptoms.

However, a study of over 500 people in 2013 found that some foods do appear to decrease the frequency of GERD symptoms.

These include: low-cholesterol protein sources, such as salmon, almonds, lean poultry and lentils, certain carbohydrates that occur in fruits, vegetables, potatoes, along with some whole-grain vitamin C-rich foods, such as fruits and vegetables high in fiber, magnesium, and potassium, especially berries, apples, pears, avocados, melons, peaches, and banana eggs, despite their fiber-rich fruits and vegetables.

Yogurt can be part of GERD's holistic dietary approach.

A comprehensive plan for GERD treatment must consider additional factors beyond the necessary changes in diet.

Restore balance to the bacterial flora in the intestines can be beneficial for many people with digestive problems. Eating fermented and pre-biotic foods could help make this happen.

In those foods, people call the bacteria probiotics. Probiotics can minimize digestive disorders by calming the entire digestive system. Prebiotics are fiber-rich foods that selectively grow beneficial bacteria.

Foods containing natural probiotics like yogurt kefir raw sauerkraut raw kimchee fresh fermented pickles and vegetables kombucha, a fermented tea drink Prebiotic-rich food. Jerusalem artichokes chicory root fiber or inulin greener banana onions garlic leeks apples the symptoms of probiotic and prebiotic foods may be reduced. Probiotics help fight a bacterial strain known as Helicobacter pylori, which may be related to GERD, some scientists believe. It needs further work to be verified.

4.4 Foods to Eat for Evading Acid Reflux Every day

Food is one of life's greatest joys, but as we've all experienced at one time or another, eating certain foods can give you discomfort. This is particularly true if you are sensitive to specific ingredients, textures or flavors, or tend to eat super-fast. A particularly unpleasant (and can be painful) food-related irritation is acid reflux, or heartburn, which occurs (ahem) when food is not well digested. "As the sphincter weakens changes in pressure cause the stomach's acidic contents to rise into the esophagus." Working into your diet with low-acid drinks and food can help you get ahead of any possible reflux situations.

Bananas & Melon

In general, eating low-acid foods and drinks will be the name of the game in terms of eating to prevent acid reflux— and that includes berries. According to the Cleveland Clinic, avoiding citrus or any other acidic fruit can help prevent acid reflux. In comparison, bananas and melons are lower in acid, which means they are less likely to trigger symptoms of acid reflux, according to Dr. Jamie Kaufman, who has recommended these fruits to The New York Times.

Oatmeal

Some decent foods with a low acidity? Throw some of the bananas into your oatmeal. The classic cereal breakfast has a pH of 7.2, the New York Times reports, making it a very neutral contribution to your day (no pun intended). Oatmeal can quickly go down and keep you full for hours to come. It can also aid with other digestive functions, with one 2005 study showing that acid reflux poop benefited babies cope with oatmeal. The more you know the better!

RECIPE#47 BROILED CHICKEN KABOBS

This heartburn-friendly recipe is easy to prepare and takes up to 35 minutes to make. An added plus is it has a low-fat content.

Because too much fat in a meal can cause heartburn, a low-fat recipe is more likely to lessen the risk of heartburn. So now, without fear, you can indulge your passion for kabobs

This recipe requires soaked wooden skewers, but some kabob pundits prefer to use metal skewers to avoid the chance that the wood will split into the food. It's your choice. Before using, lightly coat the skewers with a small amount of olive oil. The grain falls into them much more quickly.

Ingredients:

1 teaspoon of olive oil

1 teaspoon of oregano

1 teaspoon of basil

1/2 teaspoon of rosemary

1/2 teaspoon of parsley

1 1/2 pounds of boneless chicken breast each into1-inch pieces Non-stick vegetable cooking spray

4 cups of rosemary cut into1-inch pieces

3 cups of whole-button mushrooms, stalks removed

1 cup of long-grain brown rice, cooked under the desperate need for cooking;

Directions:

1. Combine 1 spoonful of olive oil, 1 teaspoon of oregano, 1 teaspoon basil, 1/2 teaspoon of rosemary and 1/2 teaspoon of parsley in a medium bowl.

2. Apply 1.5 pounds of chicken pieces to a bowl and mix well, covering the chicken on all sides.

3. Let them sit for five minutes.

4. Spray non-stick vegetable spray on a broiler saucepan.

5. In the bowl of the chicken mixture stir 4 cups of zucchini pieces and 3 cups of button mushrooms until well coated.

6. Alternating thread chicken, mushrooms, and zucchini bits, on all 8 skewers.

7. Place the kabobs on Pan broiler. Broil to each hand for 5 minutes, turning once. Hot brown rice to serve.

Note: Traditionally kabobs are served over a rice bed, with pita bread. They may be served with dipping sauces of choice on or off the skewer.

Fun Fast Facts about Kabobs

A shish kebab is a grilled meat skewer (lamb, beef, chicken and pork in some crops) with vegetables such as green peppers, onions and mushrooms. Pronounced kabob, kebab, kebob or kebab, the term comes from the Turkish language.

Almond Milk

According to a gastroenterologist Prevention from almond milk help get rid of acid reflux which is occurring due to its essential nutrients. the ability to alkalinize the body allows it to thrive in a proper state.

Cow's milk can sometimes contribute to reflux, so almond milk is a great substitution. Almond milk is alkaline— the opposite of acidic — that helps fight acid reflux. Drink plain or add after a meal to smoothies.

Greek Yogurt

Greek yogurt, skier, or kefir with healthy gut strains that promote bacteria and probiotics have been shown to help prevent acid reflux.

"Foods with healthy bacteria [such as yogurt] can help to improve digestion and reduce the acid reflux frequency," nutritionist Lisa Hugh told Bustle earlier. Have a breakfast yogurt or a snack. It's packed with other essential nutrients and protein too!

Licorice

Like ginger, licorice is a long-touched herbal heartburn remedy. A 2014 review of case reports showed that deglycyrrhizinated licorice as part of a broader integrative approach helps children control acid reflux. (Deglycyrrhizinated means that a substance linked to high blood pressure has been removed.) This can be picked up at the pharmacy in tablet form.

Fennel

If you don't like the licorice taste, you probably won't like the fennel taste but know that both of these bitterly sweet herbs can help with acid reflux. Fennel has powerful abilities to help soothe the process of stomach and digestion, and reduce acidity. For best results, take fennel as part of a salad or after a meal.

Lean Protein

While foods with a higher fat content are not necessarily "bad" to you— avocados, for example, are shock-full— fat can exacerbate reflux of acid. Choosing lean protein sources like lean meats, beans, legumes, and low-fat dairy will help avoid reflux when higher in fat proteins is replaced.

Flavored Gum

Chewing gum help surprisingly manage reflux; it promotes the production of saliva, and saliva, which is low in acid, helps to soothe your irritated esophagus, according to Harvard Health. However, spearmint or peppermint may trigger acid reflux, Cochrane says, so sticking to fruit-flavored gum or another more neutral flavor is better.

Ginger

According to Harvard Health, Ginger has been used for decades as a natural remedy for acid reflux, GERD, and heartburn. The science about its effects on heartburn is so: a 2019 review of the effects of ginger on digestion found that while ginger had positive impact on nausea, one of its rare side effects was heartburn. Nonetheless, the study concluded that for nausea and other digestive problems "ginger could be considered a harmless and probably successful choice" and that more research is needed, so if ginger helps you, more power for you. Eat plain with a meal or toss it into a veggie dish. You can also throw a few in a juice, water, or smoothie and after eating, take a few sips.

RECIPE#48 EASY OVERNIGHT OATMEAL

If you often rush out of the door in the morning, it may be challenging to imagine waking up early to cook a healthy breakfast! You may grab a not - so-healthy one in the office break room through a drive-thru window or rely on donuts, or you may skip breakfast altogether. A healthy breakfast has proven its benefits: more energy, better focus, maintaining a healthier weight, and the list continues. So why is it so hard to do it?

It shouldn't be! With this simple overnight oatmeal recipe, all it takes is five minutes before you go to bed to have a nutritious morning breakfast ready to go. Filling whole grain oats, smooth Greek yogurt, and fruit make this a delicious and nutritious meal that can be enjoyed either cold or dry, and the flavor choices are endless so you never get bored.

Ingredients:

1/2 cup skim milk with 1/4 cup plain Greek yogurt, 1 teaspoon honey and 1/2 cup of vanilla rolled oats, 1/2 cup of any fruit

Directions:

1.   In a jar with a lid, whisk together the milk, yogurt, honey and vanilla. Stir in some oats. Cover and refrigerate it overnight.

2.   Stir in your favorite fruit in the morning, and enjoy.

3.   I like to keep my overnight oatmeal simple with a little vanilla and honey, but don't hesitate to add any spices or flavors you might think of. Cinnamon, berries, nuts, and seeds all are great ways to spice up this meal!

4.   For a meal that is diabetes friendly, omit the honey and instead use one packet of stevia.

5.   Are sure to use certified gluten-free oats to make this gluten-free.

6.   Heat up 60 to 90 seconds in the microwave to serve hot, stirring halfway through. You can make two or three jars at once so that breakfast is available in a few days ' worth.

RECIPE#49 TOMATO SAUCE-FREE LASAGNA

Total Time: 60 min Prep Time: 25 min Cook Time: 35 min
Servings: 10

Nutrition Highlights (by serving): 314 calories 10g fat 32 g
carbs 22 g protein

Do you love lasagna but tomato-based products cause
heartburn? Now, with this low-fat, no tomato sauce lasagna
recipe, you can enjoy this Italian classic-with a bit of a twist.
Instead of a traditional red pasta sauce, this recipe focuses
on lean ground beef, beef broth, low-fat mozzarella cheese,
and a creamy homemade low-fat Alfredo. That makes for a
slightly different but delicious lasagna for which the entire
family will beg.

This recipe is low in fat as a bonus–lean ground beef, low-
fat cream cheese, skim milk and fresh mozzarella cheese
make a rich, nutritious yet healthy comfort dish.

Ingredients:

12 ounces wide lasagna noodles 12 ounces very lean
ground beef (ground round or ground sirloin) Non-stick
cooking spray 1/2 cup low-sodium beef broth 1/4 cup low-

fat cream cheese 1 1/4 cup skim milk, split 1 table cup all-purpose flour 2 table cup butter or 1/2 cup margarine shredded good-quality Parmesan cheese salt and freshly ground pepper cheese

Directions:

1. Put salted water on to boil and cook the noodles until they are tender. Drain well.

2. Add the browned beef and beef broth in a large bowl. Only fire together.

3. Combine the cream cheese, 1/4 cup milk, and flour in a medium mixing bowl. Beat until it blends well. Pour in the remaining 1 cup of skim milk and beat to shape the sauce until smooth.

4. Melt butter over medium heat into a large, non-stick saucepan. Remove the milk-cream cheese mixture and continue to heat until the sauce has thickened for about 4 minutes, stirring constantly.

5. Add salt and pepper to taste in Parmesan cheese.

6. Add 1 cup of Alfredo low-fat sauce to the bottom of a 13x9-inch baking pan. Add 3 lasagna noodle strips and spread half of the beef mixture over the top.

7. Lay down a further 3 lasagna noodle plates. Spread the beef mixture over the top and lay the remaining 3 lasagna noodle strips.

8.   Spread Alfredo sauce very top with the remaining 1 cup low-fat. Sprinkle with mozzarella cheese, and bake until bubbly and golden for 25 to 35   minutes.

RECIPE#50 LOW-FAT SHRIMP WITH PASTA

Nutrition Highlights (by serving)

399 calories 9 g fat 50 g carbs 28 g protein

This quick and easy pasta shrimp takes just 25 minutes to prepare from beginning to end. Combining shrimp with other low-fat ingredients makes this a shrimp and pasta recipe that can be enjoyed even by people who experience heartburn, because high-fat foods are known to cause heartburn. It's a perfect candidate for a busy weekend dinner, or it can easily transition into a company-worthy meal with a salad and a baguette of crusty bread.

Ingredients

Non-stick vegetable spray

1 tablespoon of olive oil

2 teaspoons of dried basil

1/2 teaspoon of salt

1 teaspoon of dried oregano

1 pound of medium shrimp

8 ounces of uncooked angel hair pasta

1/2 cup of grated

Parmesan cheese

Direction:

1.   Set the pasta in a pot of water to boil.

2.   Coat a large skillet with non-stick spray for cooking vegetables lightly. Place on medium to high heat, and then add olive oil. Let it run for around 1 to 2 minutes.

3.   Add dried basil, salt, shrimp and dried oregano. Toss to coat herbal shrimps and cook for 6 to 8 minutes, or until the shrimp is cooked and turns pink once.

4.   While, cook the pasta according to the instructions of the package. Wash and wash.

5.   Toss a mixture of shrimp and hot pasta.

6.   Sprinkle with and top with Parmesan cheese.

How to Peel and Devein Shrimp

If the head is still attached and you want it removed, twist it gently. Then, starting at the head end, go below where the legs are mounted, and peel off the legs and shell. If you want to leave that tail on, go ahead. Otherwise, holding on to the shrimp's body, remove the rear with a soft tug.

Lay down the shrimp and cut along the middle of the back of the shrimp with a paring knife to expose the vein. Try not to cut too deeply, and take the thin gray thread out. Remove the shell as directed above for tail-on shrimp but keep the last segment attached and then devein. Rinse the shrimp and pat dry before adding them to your favorite recipe.

Aloe

Think of aloe Vera as a gel that is used to treat sunburn, but the anti-inflammatory effects that make it a soothing post-holiday skin treatment also make the plant useful in managing acid reflux. A randomized control found it to be safe and well tolerated and reduced the frequencies of all the GERD symptoms assessed. pick it up from most supermarkets as a juice.

When you have signs of acid reflux it may be a good idea to change your food choices so that after a delicious meal you can feel better and more relaxed. eating gradually, eating smaller, more frequent meals throughout the day and waiting for a minimum of three hours before lying down. But in the end, if acid reflux gets in the way you live your life, you should talk to your doctor that how to manage it.

If you notice that any home remedies are increasingly needed to manage reflux symptoms, it's time to talk to a doctor regarding what you can do to manage those symptoms better. Uncontrolled reflux can damage the esophagus and increase the risk of further health problems over time.

4.5 Natural Remedies

Other natural treatments that may ease the symptoms of GERD include deglycyrrhized liquor ice; ginger and slippery elm bark which reduce symptoms such as relieve nausea and improve gastric emptying.

Slippery elm contains elevated mucilage levels. Mucilage can coat the throat and soothe the stomach. It may also cause mucus to be secreted by the stomach, which helps protect it against acid damage.

2010 BMC Gastroenterology research suggests an oral melatonin supplement may also be useful in treating GERD symptoms. The researchers, however, recommend this only as one aspect of the treatment, and further studies are needed to validate these findings.

it is suggested that weight loss and head rising during sleep can minimize GERD symptoms. While people usually think that GERD is a chronic disorder, it doesn't have to be permanent.

RECIPE#51 HEALTHIER DEVILED EGGS

A basic recipe with a healthy twist. The reduced mayonnaise and sugar-free sweet taste take what is usually high in calories, fat, sugar, and carbohydrates and turn this recipe into an appetizer that you can enjoy without feeling guilty about. You can also add herbs, low-fat blue cheese dressing or even crab or smoked salmon to vary the flavors.

This recipe requires a sugar-free sweet taste, but you can leave it out, or use dill pleasure. add bit of sugar for balancing flavor.

Ingredients

12 big, hard-cooked eggs

1/4 cup of reduced-fat mayonnaise

2 table spoons of prepared mustard (yellow or brown)

1/4 cup of dill (optional)

A few drops of hot sauce

1/4 teaspoon of kosher salt

Ground black pepper to taste

2 table spoons of fresh chives (optional)

Sprinkle of paprika

Directions:

1.   Peel the eggs then split them carefully into half and transfer the yolks to a medium bowl.

2.   Mix the egg yolks well with a fork, and the remaining ingredients together well.

3.   Fill the egg white halves cavities, smooth the mixture over the top (or you can use a pastry bag to pip it in).

4.   Sprinkle on top with extra paprika. Refrigerate to ready for serving.

RECIPE#52 LOW-CALORIE CREAMY COLESLAW

Total Time: 15 min Prep Time: 15 min Cook Time: 0 min
Servings: 7 (1 cup each)

Nutrition Highlights (by serving)

74 calories 4 g fat 6 g carbs 3 g protein

We know an easy way to cut down on calories and fat in coleslaw is to swap the creamy dressing to a vinegar-based one. Because mayonnaise is the culprit, this is the ingredient to be substituted for. When mixing a reduced-fat mayo with Greek nonfat yogurt, you retain the creamy texture of the coleslaw and a little of the mayonnaise flavor. However, if the result is too tangy, add a bit of sugar to balance it. Use a seasoning mix such as Penney's buttermilk ranch seasoning to make that coleslaw dressing even faster. This coleslaw with a barbecue or any grilled food is excellent. The cold creaminess up against hot BBQ spices is perfect.

Ingredients:

- 1/3 cup of mayonnaise fat
- 2/3 cup of Greek non-fat yogurt
- 2 teaspoons of lemon juice (freshly squeezed)
- 1 teaspoon of garlic powder

- 1 teaspoon of onion powder

- 1/8 teaspoon of paprika

- 1/4 teaspoon of black pepper

- 1/4 teaspoon of salt

- 1 pound of chopped sugar, shredded or 1 bag of coleslaw mix

Directions:

1. In a liquid measuring cup, mix the mayonnaise, yogurt, lemon juice, and seasonings.

2. The lemon juice, salt, and sugar are tasted and balanced to your taste.

3. Place the cod in a large bowl and pour over the dressing. To make it easier, you might want to mix half of the cabbage and stuffing at a time.

RECIPE#53 BAKED FRENCH FRIES

Fried foods are often what those who encounter heartburn often neglect. Instead of greasy French fries, it is better to switch to a baked version for symptoms and it slashes the fat and calories.

At nearly 400 calories and 17 grams of fat per serving a medium order of fast-food fries comes in. This recipe comes with just 194 calories and 4 grams of fat. Say hello to crunchy chips, and bye-bye to flare ups from heartburn.

Ingredients:

• 4 medium russet potatoes

• 1 spoon of olive oil

• 1/2 spoon of kosher salt

• 1/4 spoon of freshly ground black pepper

Directions:

1. Oven preheats to 400F.

2. Line a parchment paper baking sheet, and set aside.

3.   Scrub potatoes well, leaving the skins on to remove any dirt.

4.   Slice into large slices long by long.

5.   Again, cut into sticks of even thickness.

6.   Transfer to baking sheet prepared.

7.   Add olive oil with salt and pepper to taste.

8.   Toss well to have the seasoning distributed.

9.   Bake 35 to 40 minutes, during the cooking, tossing once or twice.

10.   Remove from the oven when golden and crisp, and allow cooling down slightly before serving.

Leave the skin on the potatoes to take advantage of the vitamins and minerals contained therein. To add a kick of seasonal flavor with chili powder, herbal salt, or even a few dried thyme shakes. Slice into fries and store in a bowl of cold water to prevent the potatoes from turning brown, if you want to prepare the vegetables in advance. When made to bake drain and pat dry before being put on the sheet plane.

Lining the pan with parchment paper not only makes it easy to clean, but when using a small amount of oil, it stops the potatoes from falling in.

If tomatoes trigger symptoms of heartburn for you, you should control the amount of ketchup or barbecue sauce in which you dip these fries in — a few tablespoons max should be enough. If you want to altogether avoid these sauces, instead opt for a little guacamole. Keep controlled portion here too. Although avocados add healthy fats to your side, for some, the creaminess may also trigger heartburn. Hummus or a little yogurt sauce makes great dips too.

RECIPE#54 WHOLE GRAIN WILD BLUEBERRY MUFFINS

A blueberry muffin is an apparently innocent breakfast from its name's sound. How could something be unhealthy with a seed, right? Sadly, most blueberry muffins are just glorified cupcakes twice the size, so if you're craving a bread your best bet is to make yourself a bunch. These whole grain wild blueberry muffins are made for extra fiber with whole wheat flour, and tasty wild blueberries with less sugar for sweetness. They're great to go for breakfast alongside some fruit and yogurt or eggs. If your morning is chaotic, they're easy to grab in the morning on your way out of the door. One batch makes 12 muffins, allowing you to freeze half of them for later.

Ingredients:

- 1 1/2 cups + 2 tablespoons of white whole wheat flour, split

- 1/2 cup of sugar

- 1/2 tablespoon of baking powder (low sodium if possible)

- 1 tablespoon of lemon zest

- 1 cup of almond milk

- 1/4 cup of unfit Greek yogurt

- 2 large eggs

- 2 teaspoons of vanilla extract

- 1 cup of frozen wild blueberries

Directions:

1.   Oven heat to 400F. Sprinkle with a cooking spray or line with muffin liners a regular muffin tin, and then spray with the cooking spray.

2.   Whisk the flour, sugar, baking powder, and lemon zest in a large bowl for 1 1/2 cups.

3.   Whisk wet ingredients together into a separate bowl. Pour in dry ingredients and stir gently until just mixed together.

4.   Toss blueberries in bowl along with 2 tablespoons of flour left over. Fold in softly into the batter.

5.   Scoop batter into muffin and fill 3/4 of the way. Bake until clean comes to a toothpick inserted in the middle. Remove muffins from the pan 10 minutes before cooling.

Fresh blueberries or standard frozen blueberries can be substituted for this. Apply 2 teaspoons of lemon zest to the batter to make lemon blueberry muffins.

To keep these muffins, lower in sodium, I left out the salt and baking soda as in most baked goods these are excellent sources of sodium. If you can find low sodium baking powder, it would make sodium baking powder even lower, but it also works regularly.

As with any muffins, stir the batter into the blueberries until it is just moistened and folds very gently to keep the cupcakes light and airy. Mixing over will produce denser, more healthy muffins.

RECIPE#55 LEMON-ZESTER SHRIMP ON AVOCADO TOAST

A balanced dinner does not take long to prepare. Some days, a few pantry and fridge staples can be thrown together for a quick but elegant meal. Such staples include creamy heart-healthy fats, filling fiber, and flavorful protein in this recipe.

Even if you experience heartburn you can enjoy creamy foods. For starters, the avocados make a good stand-in for spreads and sauces. The secret to this is the management of parts. Lemon zest is used to season the shrimps. Although citrus-rich lemon juice will cause reflux, it is unlikely that the punch would, so you can use it to get a similar flavor profile.

Ingredients:

- 8 medium shrimp
- 1/2 teaspoon of olive oil
- 1/2 teaspoon of lemon zest
- 1/8 teaspoon of cumin
- 1 teaspoon of cilantro, finely chopped
- 2 slices of wheat bread
- 1/2 medium avocado, mashed

- pinch of salt
- 1/4 of mango

Directions:

1.   Combine the shrimp in a small bowl with olive oil, lemon zest, cumin and optional cilantro.

2.   Heat over medium heat a small frying pan, and add the shrimp. Cook for 4 to 5 minutes and flip halfway through.

3.   While the shrimp cooks, toast the whole slices of wheat bread and mash the avocado with the salt.

4.   Spread the mashed avocado on toasted bread and top with slices of mango, then shrimp.

You can also look for a source of protein other than shrimp, Low sodium turkey or chicken deli slices would pair the avocado well, and mango is even faster!

If you have that meal on the lighter side, round it out with a side salad. Keep in mind, though, that minor portions can help prevent heartburn. Lighter fiber and protein-rich meals can help to reduce your overall calorie intake, thus helping with weight loss. Being at a healthy weight takes away the pressure from your stomach, which research has shown can help ease the symptoms of acid reflux.

Chapter 5: Your food, your healer!

GERD diet is a vital treatment part of both occasional Heartburn, also called acid reflux and the more chronic gastro esophageal reflux disease. The menu focuses on the elimination of foods that reduce the stress of the esophageal sphincter (LES), delay gastric emptying, and increase the risk of stomach acid flowing to your esophagus.

No single-size GERD diet, so it is essential that you experiment with the menu to identify and remove food that triggers your chest or throat burning sensation.

GERD occurs when the sphincter muscles at the bottom of your esophagus become weak and relax if not. It causes fluid from your abdomen to return to your throat, causing symptoms such as Heartburn, cough, and swallowing problems. GERD can lead to vomiting, respiratory problems, reduced esophagus, and increased risk of esophageal cancer in more severe cases1. GERD helps your muscle sphincter lower esophageal and stays closed after you eat so you will have fewer of these problems.

To achieve this, the GERD diet concentrates on preventing foods that have been shown to trigger reflux and symptoms more frequently. These are primarily acidic and high-fat foods (note, however, that eliminating food causes will not guarantee GERD management).

Besides the increase in stomach acid, high-fat meals delay gastric emptying and lead to acid reflux in the lower esophagus. Very acidic foods can irritate your stomach and esophagus in particular.

It is also advisable to increase fiber. Higher fiber diets increased the pressure of the esophageal sphincter, reduced the number of acids assisted, and reduced the number of heartburn occurrences. To test the theories, scientists called on people with Heartburn to add 15 g of a phylum fiber supplement daily — and it worked.3 In a 2016 study published in Diseases of the esophagus, it was found that eating the diet in a Mediterranean way is associated with a lower risk of GERD.

This way of eating will lead to some weight loss in addition to improving the symptoms. Overweight means you run a significantly higher GERD risk, and a lot of research has shown that weight loss is one of the best ways to prevent the condition. Reduced weight of 10 percent improves GERD symptoms and frequently permits people to go away from prescribed acid blocker drugs

(with their doctor's approval).4 The National Health Institutes and the American College of Gastroenterology are recommending a diet-first approach to the treatment of GERD.

Non-Compliant Foods

Whole and cracked grains. Fatty dairy products or non-dairy products. Lean meats (such as lean beef, skinless chicken, seafood).Whole soy foods (e.g., tofu or tempeh) lens, pigment, and other legumes; Healthy fats such as olive trees.

Compliant Foods

Fruit (some exceptions) Fatty meats (e.g., lean beef, skinless chicken, seafood), Besides the choice of more compliant foods and the elimination or reduction of non-compliant ones, it is essential to monitor your servings, mainly if you are overweight.

Recommended Timing

Your dinner at night is the most important meal to time correctly. Consider eating dinner at least two to three hours before bed, avoid some snacking late in the night and stand upright until you go to bed.6 Gravity will help you digest your food faster and reduce the risk of your diet and acid in your stomach dragging your bottom esophagus while you sleep.

It is not essential to have your meals or to eat them on a schedule, but instead of bigger ones, it is essential to eat small foods. Large meals generate more stomach acid, take more time to digest, and put extra pressure on your low esophagus.

Instead of eating three big meals, you may feel better if you consume and spread five small meals so that they are digested before eating again.

For healthier food, fewer calories, and less fat, use healthy cooking practices, including sauté, grilling, roasting, braising, or baking.

Cooking Tips

Stop frying deeply. If you lack the crispy crunch of fried food, try an air fryer that only uses a little oil.

Store your cupboard or refrigerator by the above list so that you are ready to serve as a substitute for hot spices, onions, and garlic.

The GERD diet can and should be very flexible except those foods that are to be avoided. This and any diet is essential to work with your lifestyle, so feel free to include more food and pay attention to how it affects your symptoms.

Experiment with new foods and flavors to replace anything you lack. The GERD diet could only open up a wholly new and safer way to eat.

The GERD diet is indeed an excellent diet for everyone because it stresses higher nutrition, less fatty foods, and smaller food, all of which will help you keep your weight healthy.

Its emphasis on a Mediterranean diet and the fiber-rich dietary pattern is consistent with the U.S. Dietary Guidelines 2015-2020. Health and Human Services Department and the U.S. Agriculture. If you travel and have limited options for food, or if your friends or family have a specific love for pepperoni or pad Thai, it might be difficult for you to follow a GERD diet. If you don't cook to yourself, it could be helpful to discuss your diet objectives with friends and family and have a plan for what you will eat in advance.

For all people, foods on the "safe" list may not be the same. Similarly, some might need to avoid those you can tolerate. Eventually, you will have to follow the diet in a structured way for at least a few weeks and note the items that seem to enhance or intensify the symptoms.

RECIPE#56 APPLE RAISIN FLAPJACKS

Start your day off right at breakfast with these delicious apple flapjacks.

Ingredients:

3 Egg whites along with Fat-free milk, 1 cup Reduced fat buttermilk, 2 cup apples (peeled, cored, and heavily chopped) Raisins, 1 cup Nutmeg, 1/2 teaspoon

Directions:

1.   Whisk up to foamy whites in large bowl. Whisk in milk and stir in baking mixture.

2.   Add ingredients left over. The only mix to blend.

3.   Heat medium-heat griddle or large skillet; brush with vegetable spray. Portion batter on the grid with a measure of 1/4 cup.

4.   Cook until well browned, turning once, at each side for about 3 minutes.

5.   Serve with fresh maple syrup or non-fat yogurt.

RECIPE#57 TURKEY, GREEN BEAN AND ALMOND SAUTÉ

Ingredients:

oil, 2 + 1 teaspoon Boneless turkey breast, 1/2-pound 1 celery stalk, Green beans, 1 cup Cornstarch, one teaspoon Reduced sodium soy sauce, 2 tablespoons Garlic powder, 1/4 teaspoon Slivered almonds, 2 tablespoons

Directions:

1.   Fix this turkey, green bean and white rice almond as aside. Heat 2 teaspoons Add the turkey strips and cook for 4-5 minutes until well done. Transfer to a plate and put it away.

2.   Add a further spoonful of oil to the pan. Add celery and green beans, and then cook for 2-3 minutes until tender-crisp.

3.   Reduce heat to low, and bring turkey back to pan. Mix the cornstarch, soy sauce, and garlic powder and add to the pan. Cook for 1-2 minutes until sauce thickens.

4.   Sprinkle, and serve with almonds.

RECIPE#58 BAKED PORK LOIN CHOPS OVER VEGETABLES

Taste these baked pork loin chops with stomach-friendly herbs and vegetables!

Ingredients:

Boneless pork loin chops (about 1 big chop), 1/2-pound salt, 1/4 teaspoon Provence herbs, 1/2 teaspoon olive oil, 2 teaspoons 1/2 mid-summer squash, 1/2 sliced medium zucchini, sliced Shredded part-skim mozzarella, 1/4 cup

Directions:

1.   Preheat oven to 425 F.

2.   Slice pork half lengthwise and cross-section ally, so you end up with 4 pieces from 1 chop. Season with the salt, then sprinkle with Provence herbs.

3.   Coat the olive oil in a baking dish, then add the squash and zucchini.

4.   Top each party with pork squash and zucchini. Sprinkle with mozzarella, and then bake 15-20 minutes in the oven until the pork is cooked through.

RECIPE#59 BROCCOLI FRITTATA

A new twist to your morning eggs-a frittata broccoli.

Ingredients:

Non-fat cottage cheese, 1/2 cup of dried dill, 1/2 cup of fat-free egg substitute, 2 cups of broccoli, 2 cups of oil, 1 teaspoon of margarine, 2 spoons of 1 large onion, diced

Directions:

1.   Mix cottage cheese and egg substitute; set aside.

2.   In a large non-stick frying pan, sauté onions over medium heat in oil for 5 minutes, or until tender.

3.   Add broccoli and dill; sauté 5 minutes, or soften the broccoli mixture. Set aside vegetables.

4.   Wipe frying casserole. Add 1 teaspoon of margarine to spread and swirl over the pan.

5.   Add half the vegetable mixture, then add half the egg mixture; lift and rotate the pan so that the eggs are distributed evenly.

6.   Lift the eggs around the edges so that uncooked portions can flow beneath them.

7. Turn the heat to medium, cover the saucepan and cook until set to top.

8. Invert onto a serving plate and wedge-cut.

9. Repeat with the remaining teaspoon of margarine, a mixture of vegetables and eggs.

RECIPE#60 PENNE WITH SHRIMP AND SPINACH

Ingredients:

Penne pasta, 4 ounces of olive oil, 1 table spoon medium or sizeable uncooked shrimp, peeled and deveined, 1/2-pound
A dash of Basil garlic powder, chopped, 2 table spinach
Baby spinach, 4 cups of Parmesan cheese, 2 table spoons

Directions:

1.   Cook pasta al dente according to the instructions of the package. Reserve 1/2 cup of water when pasta is done, and drain the rest.

2.   Heating oil over medium heat in a non-stick skillet.

3.   Shrimp on top and cook for minute. Then, turn over the shrimp and add the basil and garlic. Cook 1-2 more minutes, until the shrimp is cooked through.

4.   Fill the skillet with spinach, pasta and reserved cooking water and mix until the spinach is just wilted.

5.   Parmesan cheese on top.

5.1 Sore Throat and Acid Reflux

Anybody can occasionally experience Heartburn or acid reflux. However, if you experience it more than two or more times a week, you may be at risk for complications that could affect your throat's health.

Learn about regular heartburn complications and how you can protect your throat against damage.

How GERD can harm the esophagus

This burning sensation is stomach acid that is harmful to the skin's lining. Repeated exposure of the stomach acid to the esophagus lining can cause the so-called esophagitis over time.

Esophagitis is an inflammation that is likely to cause injuries such as erosion, ulcers and scar tissue. Esophagitis symptoms can include pain, swallowing difficulty, and more acid regurgitation.

A doctor can use the combination of tests, including upper endoscopy and biopsy to diagnose this condition.

If you have been diagnosed with esophagitis, your doctor will probably start treatment immediately because an inflamed esophagus can lead to more complications of your health.

GERD and esophagitis Complications When GERD and esophagitis symptoms are not managed; your stomach acid can continue to damage your esophagus. Repeated damage may over time lead to the following complications:

Esophagus narrowing, which is called esophageal serenity and can be caused by GERD-based scar tissue or tumors. It can be difficult for you to swallow or to catch food in your throat.

Esophageal rings: these are unusual tissue rings or folds that appear in the lower part of the esophagus. Such tissue bands can restrict the throat and cause swallowing problems.

Esophagi of Barrett: this is a condition in which cells in the lining of the esophagus are damaged by acid in the stomach and become similar to those in the cells lining the intestine. You may experience no symptoms; this is a rare condition but it may increase your risk of developing esophageal cancer. Through proper treatment for persistent Heartburn or GERD, all three of these symptoms can be prevented.

How Acid Reflux and GERD can damage the throat

Apart from potentially damaging the lower esophagus, the common cardiovascular or GERD tears the upper throat as well. This can happen if the stomach acid enters the back of your throat or nasal respiratory tract. Laryngopharyngeal reflux (LPR) is often referred to as the condition.

LPR is also sometimes referred to as a "silent reflux" because symptoms that people easily recognize do not always present. It is essential to check LPR for people with GERD to prevent possible throat or voice damage. Symptoms of LPR can consist of the following:

- hoarseness
- chronic throat clearing
- feeling "pin" in your throat
- persistent cough or cough waking you from sleep
- shaking episodes
- "rawness" in your throat
- voice problems (especially in singers or professional vocals)

Prevention of future damage

No matter if you are experiencing frequent heartbeat, GERD, LPR or combination. Talk to your doctor and make the following lifestyle

Eat smaller food more often and take your time to chew. Avoid excessive consumption. Increase overweight physical activity. Growing your dietary fiber. Increase your diet of fruit and vegetables. Stay upright after meals for at least one hour. Avoid eating 2 to 3 hours in advance of bedtime. Avoid activating foods such as high fat and sugar, alcohol, caffeine and chocolate. Keep weight healthy. Stop smoking. Raise the bed head six inches.

RECIPE #61 BANANA PORK LOIN

This rare banana pork loin puts together two heartburn-friendly ingredients for an exciting new meal.

Ingredients:

2 teaspoons Boneless pork loin, oil, 1/2-pound 1 Large banana, sliced Curry powder*, 1/4 cup Crème fraise, 2 teaspoons

Directions:

1.   Heat canola oil over medium - high heat in a medium to large skillet. Stir in pork and sauté for 4 to 5 minutes. Remove the pig, and keep the foil warm.

2.   Slice the banana into your skillet while cooking for minute. Season the banana with the curry and add the fraise in the cream.

3.   Reduce heat to medium-low, and cook. Then stir in the pork, cover and cook for another 2 minutes.

4.   Curry powder may be triggering Heartburn (because it contains other spices such as cayenne pepper). Use it sparingly to see if it is a threat to you.

RECIPE #62 COUSCOUS SAUTÉD WITH ZUCCHINI

Couscous sautéed with zucchini and corn make an exceptionally delicious meal for burn-sensitive stomachs.

Ingredients:

couscous, olive oil, 2 teaspoons zucchini, cut into 1⁄4 by 1⁄2-inch strips Shredded carrots, 1⁄2 cup A dash of onion powder Fresh or thawed frozen corn kernels, 1⁄2 cup Salt, 1⁄4 teaspoon.

Directions:

1.   Cook couscous as directed by the package, omitting salt and fat. Deposit back.

2.   Heat the oil from medium to high heat in a large non-stick skillet. Add the corvettes, then sauté for 2 minutes. Add carrot and onion, then sauté 4-5 minutes until tender.

3.   Attach the corn and couscous, and then cook until cooked through. Season to salt.

RECIPE #63 WILD RICE AND VEGETABLE CASSEROLE

An exciting and easy wild rice and vegetable casserole using heartburn-friendly veggies and cheeses.

Ingredients:

Wild and long grain rice blend, 6 ounces of olive oil, 2 teaspoons of Brussels sprouts, trimmed and removed leaves, 2 cups of green beans, trimmed, 2 cups of salt, 1/4 teaspoon of part-skim mozzarella, shredded, 3/4 cup of goat cheese, crumbled, 4 ounces of dried cranberries, 2 table cups of walnuts, chopped, 2 table cups

Directions:

1.   Cook rice according to package

2.   In the meantime, heat oil over medium - high heat in a large, non-stick skillet. Add the sprouts and sauté over Brussels for 2-3 minutes. Cover and reduce to medium heat; cook for about 5-6 minutes, stirring occasionally, until tender. Attach the green beans and sauté, uncovered, for 2-3 minutes. Season to salt.

3.   In a baking or casserole dish, lay rice, vegetables, cheeses, walnuts and cranberries; Bake at 350 a.m. until cheese is melted for about 25 minutes.

RECIPE#64 ZUCCHINI WITH WALNUT PASTA

Ingredients

Rigatoni (or other pasta), 4 ounces of olive oil, 2 teaspoons garlic powder 1 zucchini, sliced spinach, packed, 4 cups of salt, 1/8 teaspoon of walnuts, roughly chopped, 1/4 cup

Directions:

1.   Cook pasta according to the instructions of the package, omitting salt or fat. Drain and set aside, with about 1/2 cup of pasta water reserved.

2.   In the meantime, heat 2 teaspoons of olive oil over medium-high heat in a large non-stick skillet. Add the garlic and sauté for 1-2 minutes. Add the zucchini and sauté for 3-4 minutes, until slightly golden.

3.   Turn the heat then add the spinach and drained pasta to the skillet. Toss with the zucchini and the spinach is slightly wilted until evenly distributed.

4.   Sprinkle with salt to taste. Fin, and serve with the walnuts.

RECIPE #65 ALMOND-CRUSTED CHICKEN

This delicious almond-crusted chicken uses simple ingredients to reduce your heartburn risk.

Ingredients

2 Boneless chicken breast, 1 Egg white 1/8 teaspoon salt, Parmesan cheese, 1/3 cup almonds, 1/3 cup flour, 1 tablespoon oil, 1 tablespoon

Directions:

1.   Position chicken breasts between 2 sheets of plastic wrap or wax paper and flatten with rolling pin

2.   In a shallow bowl, gently beat the egg white, and season with 1/8 teaspoon salt and pepper. Combine almonds and parmesan on a large platter.

3.   Dust the chicken breasts lightly with flour, dip in the egg, and then coat in a Parmesan mixture.

4.   Heat oil in a non-stick skillet over medium heat; Transfer chicken to skillet and cook for about 3-4 minutes, until cooked through. Mix salt and pepper with 1/8 tablespoon, and drink...

5.2 Pregnancy and Heartburn

Pregnancy and Heartburn chances are good that you are one of the female pregnant with heartburn and acid indigestion churning and burning. This generally hits somewhere in the second or third fifth, and it can be painful. Heartburn doesn't mean that your heart burns, but it's a good description of the discomfort behind your breastbone. Then it moves up to the neck and neck. Officially, gastro esophageal reflux is defined as acidic stomach juices or food and fluids go back to the esophagus. This is a hollow muscle tube between the mouth and the belly.

Why does pregnancy happen?

Most women with Heartburn never had a problem before during pregnancy. Unfortunately, you are more likely to have symptoms during pregnancy if you have Heartburn before you are pregnant. Although there are no apparent reasons for this, most experts consider that pregnancy hormones, especially progesterone, play a role. Hormones cause the esophageal sphincter to relax. It is a narrow circular muscle band at the top of the stomach. This allows partly digested food and stomach acids to return to the esophagus or reflux. Progesterone also slows down the digestive process. It keeps food longer in the stomach. Pregnancy itself — the increasing pressure of the uterus — can also play a role.

What's the problem?

Most spicy, fatty foods known to cause Heartburn are also likely to cause problems for pregnant women. During pregnancy, food does not digest or move as fast. So, eating abundant foods or overeating can also increase the risk of cardiovascular burn. It may also cause problems to eat right before bedtime. Smoking exacerbates Heartburn and is another reason to stop, particularly when pregnant.

What's better for it?

For most women, things which help reduce or prevent reflux are useful to avoid heartburn discomfort. Avoid spicy foods as well as those that contain lots of fat or grease. Many people also recommend that citrus and chocolate be avoided. Have several small meals all day long, much like' grazing,' rather than three big meals.

Some women find that between meals it is better to drink fluids instead of a meal. This can increase the amount of stomach content.

If symptoms do not improve discuss over - the-counter medicines with your healthcare provider. As chewable tablets and liquids, antacids are available. These bind the esophagus and stomach lining and neutralize stomach acid. Heartburn medicines called H2 blockers function by reducing the stomach's acid content. Although most of them, like all medicines, are considered safe during pregnancy, these should be avoided in the first trimester.

Is it going to end?

The symptoms of Heartburn tend to be mild and manageable. Ask the health care provider if you have severe Heartburn, spit blood on or bowel movements of dark color. This is a sign of your digestive system's blood. Fortunately, Heartburn usually ends with your baby's birth and your body goes back to its non-stop condition.

RECIPE#66 MOROCCAN KUMERA HASH

A hearty, cardiac breakfast with enough inbound energy to get you through the day. Perfect for brisk mornings, entertaining loved ones, or as breakfasts cooked in batch.

Ingredients:

1 big kumara 1 medium desired potato (or any other soft potato of your choice) 1 big broccoli 1 big red / green capsicum 2 big eggs 2 tsp Moroccan seasoning Olive oil

Directions:

1.   Cube kumara, potato, broccoli, and capsicum desired.

2.   Set wok on top (high) stove and frying pan (medium-high)

3.   Add olive oil to wok and fry pan

4.   Crack the eggs into the frying pan and leave until cooked

5.   Put your cubed vegetables in the wok and start stirring with wooden spoon

6.   In the vegetable mixture, mix in some Moroccan powder, stir and put the lid on, leaving for twenty seconds

7.   Repeat step 6 to step

8.   When vegetables look cooked and flavorful, remove onto the plate from wok. If not, then repeat. Place fried eggs over vegetable mixture

RECIPE#67 RICE PUDDING

Ingredients:

2 cups of cooked rice with 2 cups of rice milk 1/2 cup of granulated sugar Pinch of cooking salt Cinnamon spray (only if tolerated)

Directions:

Preheat the oven to 350 degrees. Spray the cooking spray on a bread-sized glass baking dish. Stir the rice, milk, sugar and salt into a mixing bowl. Pour into the saucepan. You want the rice to be protected by the liquid so you may need to add more milk depending on how much the rice is absorbent. Put in the oven. Remove and stir after 15 minutes, then add a little more milk if needed. Go back to the oven for 20 minutes. Remove, allow to cool and then cool. Serve the cold in cups or bowls .for dessert. Sprinkle with the cinnamon (if tolerated) before serving.

RECIPE#68 DREAMY MANGOSMOOTHIE

Research shows that drinking alcohol above the prescribed U.S. dietary guidelines increases the risk of esophageal cancer considerably. This smoothie is delicious and just as enjoyable as any drink, without the alcohol added.

Ingredients:

1 cup of coconut milk 1 splash of vanilla extract 1/2 cup of frozen mango 1/2 frozen and peeled banana

Directions:

Place the liquid first in the blender. Stir in the frozen fruit. Blend and mix until smooth. Serve in a bottle of summer cocktails.

RECIPE#69 GRILLED PLANTAINS

Plants can be both sweet and savory, a taste that transports you mentally to a tropical island. These are relatively low in sugar, and full of vitamins. They need to be very ripe when you shop for plantains, and they will appear almost black.

Ingredients:

6 Ripe plantains, peeled and horizontally cut into half-inch thick slices 1/4 cup of canola oil 1/2 cup of brown sugar Pinch of salt 2 tabs butter

Directions:

Heat grill to maximum. In a small saucepan, place the brown sugar, salt and butter and cook until the butter has melted and the sugar has dissolved. Take off heat.

Brush both sides of the plantains with oil and grill until golden brown and caramelized, for about 3 minutes per side. Remove the sugar glaze from the restaurant, and dab before eating.

RECIPE#70 SHRIMP POKE BOWLS

Poke bowls are all furious. They emerged in Hawaii and have made it to the mainland, thankfully. I was getting my first poke bowl outside New York City this summer, and now I'm addicted! While the dish usually includes raw fish, ingredients such as tofu or cooked shrimp may be used as well. My family enjoyed this version of the shrimp the whole summer.

Ingredients:

2 cups of rice, 10 peeled and cooked shrimps, 1 avocado,1/2 cucumber, 1 cup of roasted corn ,Creamy avocado dressing , 1 tabs of chia seeds for decoration The bowls are served cold, so on.

Directions:

Start by dividing the rice between two bowls when making the bowls. The base will be rice. Top with the corn, shrimp, and cucumber. Place the slices on top of avocado. Drizzle the bowls with creamy avocado dressing. Sprinkle over seeds. Serving cold.

Conclusion

Which types of recipes would a book on acid reflux help? Tums Cookies on Tacos or Pepcid AC? No, take another gander at The Food Steps to Freedom and come up with some patterns.

Some no tomato options for our top tomato dishes (and, if possible, removed the garlic and onion. If you cannot use tomato, you could use gravy rather than a marinara sauce, but that wouldn't beef stroganoff? So, we've looked at popular fatty foods in the recipes discussed and lightened them so you can eat the fried chicken!

Why is it so important to light up some of the fattiest foods in America? (Apart from the fact that food fat prevents the emptying of the stomach into the small intestine, it allows the esophageal sphincter valve to relax or weaken, and a high-fat diet promotes weight gain). When do people tend to have the most problems with acid reflux? By the time they eat out. What studies have shown that people eat a more significant amount of fat (not to mention sodium and cholesterol too). After having enjoyed a sumptuous, full meal, walk out of a restaurant complete with several rounds of dead man walking. Is that how you feel when you unleash your libations, late at night? After a beautiful meal, it is hard to enjoy the moment of pure satisfaction when you know that you are about to begin paying (big time) for your indulgences in the dining — and it doesn't mean with your credit card. For many men, after finishing their meal, the heartburn starts hitting minutes or, that might end up keeping you up all night.

To sum up the discussions, it is assumed that several medications can treat acidic reflux with a proper diet chart on the recommendation of doctors and nutritionists and that the specific heart burning friendly recipes can be followed to accelerate the healing process of healthy patients and specific GERD conditions can be treated through. Patients with severe gastro esophageal reflux disease (GERD) may choose between medication and surgery to relieve their symptoms. Still, researchers caution that while both strategies are useful, in some crucial ways they are also different.

In GERD, gastric liquids are regurgitated into the esophagus and mouth. The sour-tasting fluid often feels like it is burning as it passes, and the substances it contains, such as liver acids and bile, can inflame the esophagus and cause it damage.

In Sweden, Dr. Lars Lund ell and colleagues from Huddinge's Karolina University Hospital have studied 255 GERD cases:

One hundred twenty-two with reflux surgery and 133 with omeprazole (Prilosec) instead. Initially, the survey was intended to last for five years, but Lund ell and his team remained in regular contact with 53 surgical patients and 71 omeprazole patients after 12 years.

In Clinical Gastroenterology and Hematology researchers have reported that 28 of the 53 patients who received operation (53 percent) stayed in continuous remission (13 percent) and that "these are the safest therapies for clinical change." Of the 71 who took the medicine, 45% remained in a continuous remission with a dose adjustment and 40% remained with a fixed dose. Overall, surgery-controlled GERD symptoms such as cardiovascular disease and recurrence was more comfortable, but long-term omeprazole treatment prevented postoperative swallowing problems, flatulence, and belches or vomits incapacity.

It is noteworthy to the researchers that postoperative problems have not declined over time. Furthermore, 38% of surgical patients ultimately needed medication to minimize stomach acids. Quality-of-life ratings were "similar... in the two treatment groups throughout the entire study period.

Our hectic lifestyle triggers GERD that is usually treated with drugs that are not always so harmless. By improving our sleeping habits and preparing healthy recipes that will clean & detoxify your body, we can handle GERD the natural way.

References

1.   5 Reflux-Friendly Summer Recipes. Retrieved from https://www.healthcentral.com/article/gerd-friendly-summer-recipes

2.   GERD diet: Foods to eat and avoid. Retrieved from https://www.medicalnewstoday.com/articles/314690.php#foods-to-avoid

3.   The Best Drinks for Heartburn | Livestrong.com. Retrieved from https://www.livestrong.com/article/432019-the-best-drinks-for-heartburn/

4.   GERD Diet | Everyday Health. Retrieved from https://www.everydayhealth.com/gerd/guide/diet/

5.   11 Foods That Help Prevent Acid Reflux. Retrieved from https://www.bustle.com/p/10-foods-drinks-to-eat-to-avoid-acid-reflux-every-day-4080508

6.   Recipes. Retrieved from https://www.verywellfit.com/recipes-4157077

7.   The Best and Worst Foods When You Have Acid Reflux. Retrieved

fromhttps://www.uhhospitals.org/Healthy-at-

UH/articles/2014/04/best-and-worst-foods-for-acid-reflux

8.

        https://www.everydayhealth.com/gerd/managing/enjoy-heartburn-free-travel.aspx

9.   Recipes for People with Acid Reflux | RefluxMD. Retrieved from https://www.refluxmd.com/acid-reflux-recipes/

10.   10 Things to Stop Doing If You Have GERD. Retrieved from https://www.verywellhealth.com/stop-doing-with-gerd-1742213

11.   Gastro esophageal reflux disease (GERD) Home Remedies. Retrieved from https://www.healthline.com/health/gerd/home-remedies#herbal-remedies

12.   What You Should Know About Dairy and Acid Reflux. Retrieved from https://www.healthline.com/health/gerd/dairy-and-acid-reflux#dairy-substitutes

13.   Dr. Gourmet's Easy Guide to Eating Healthy. Retrieved from https://www.drgourmet.com/eatinghealthy/index.shtml

14.   Probiotics for Acid Reflux: Know the Facts. Retrieved from https://www.healthline.com/health/gerd/probiotics-for-acid-reflux

15.   What Is Acid Reflux Disease? Retrieved from https://www.webmd.com/heartburn-gerd/guide/what-is-acid-reflux-disease#2

Lightning Source UK Ltd.
Milton Keynes UK
UKHW020750020221
378105UK00013B/339